EUROPEAN FOUNDATION FOR TH
OF LIVING AND WORKING CONDIT

T0229403

Telematics for Health

the role of telehealth and telemedicine
in homes and communities

Marjorie Gott

RADCLIFFE MEDICAL PRESS • OXFORD and NEW YORK

OFFICE FOR OFFICIAL PUBLICATIONS OF
THE EUROPEAN COMMUNITIES • LUXEMBOURG

Published in 1995 by Radcliffe Medical Press Ltd, 15 Kings Meadow, Ferry Hinksey Road, Oxford, OX2 0DP, UK and 141 Fifth Avenue, New York, NY 10010, USA; and Office for Official Publications of the European Communities, 2, rue Mercier, L-2985 Luxembourg

Typeset by AMA Graphics Ltd, Preston, England

British Library Cataloguing in Publication Data

A catalogue record for this book is available from the British Library

ISBN 1 85775 023 3

Library of Congress Cataloging-in-Publication Data is available

Office for Official Publications of the European Communities, 2, rue Mercier, L-2985 Luxembourg

ISBN 92 826 8761 9

Catalogue No SY-85-94-575-EN-C

Publication No. EF/94/24/EN of the European Foundation for the Improvement of Living and Working Conditions, Loughlinstown House, Shankill, Co. Dublin, Ireland

Contents

Foreword

Telemedicine and telehealth – the use of telecommunications and informatics for medical and health purposes – are already growing activities in Europe. Their impact has moved beyond the research stage, and has consequences for the quality of life of European citizens.

The case studies that follow show how technology can be responsive to the health needs of individuals and communities. The key principles seem to be involvement of potential users from the beginning and a low technology approach.

The research reviews case studies from seven countries. Present recommendations are for better policy, practice and the direction of future work. Evidence is based on interviews with users, providers and managers, and captures a freshness and insights that much academic research lacks. Consequently, this book can help professionals working in the community, policy makers and health service users.

The book makes a plea for technology targeted at groups with special needs, such as the elderly, the young, the disabled and pregnant women. The author, through practical examples, highlights how technology may empower these citizens and enable them to lead better and healthier lives.

The European Foundation for the Improvement of Living and Working Conditions has been developing research in the field of new technologies and quality of life for many years. The electronic home was chosen as a framework for several research projects that assessed the social impact of telematics – the combination of telecommunications and informatics – at home. These projects have considered telework, the urban dimension of the electronic home, and telehealth and telemedicine.

We are grateful to the author, Marjorie Gott, for her enthusiasm and the high quality of her research. We would like to express our appreciation, too, to Radcliffe Medical Press and the Office for Official Publications of the European Communities for their support in making this book possible.

Clive Purkiss
Director
European Foundation
for the Improvement of
Living and Working Conditions

Eric Verborgh
Deputy Director
European Foundation
for the Improvement of
Living and Working Conditions

Preface

The purpose of this book is to examine and comment on recent trends in health care policy making and medical telematics in Europe. The author is aiming to flag a new, and potentially more rewarding, way forward that can be accessed by new technologies, but not exclusively medical ones.

It will be argued that the social technologies (television, telephone and videophone) have an important role to play in promoting the health and well-being of European citizens. To use these most effectively, however, it is necessary to revalue, and listen to, all citizens of Europe (including the young, the disabled and the elderly). It is also necessary to focus on the settings where most of life is lived: the home and the community.

This book describes some of the health promotion opportunities that can be realized through the use of modern telecommunications technologies. A review of case study experiences in seven countries is undertaken.

The study was commissioned by the European Foundation for the Improvement of Living and Working Conditions as a response to growing concern that medical technology has not been supporting Health For All principles.

Marjorie Gott

Acknowledgements

The author is grateful to the European Foundation for the Improvement of Living and Working Conditions for commissioning this work, and in particular to Jaume Costa (Research Manager, European Foundation) for his advice, encouragement and support.

She is also indebted to all the people who allowed her into their institutions and their homes, and showed her such kindness and generosity. Special thanks, however, is reserved for her partner, Brian, who has supported her whole-heartedly throughout this project, both as a business partner and a (very special) husband.

1 Health and Technology: Making Connections

'The information society can be a threat to our physical, mental and social well-being and we should learn to recognize it and treat it as a threat. That way, we might at least reduce the health effect somewhat, and learn at the same time how to enhance the potential health benefits.'

(Hancock, 1992)

Much of the 'health' work undertaken in this century has in fact been illness work. Illness work is big business; medicine coupled with telematics is even bigger business. The use of telematics in medicine is growing and the scale and scope of this growth need to be challenged.

In order to challenge the unchecked rise in the use of telematics in medical care, it is necessary to revisit and contextualize some key issues that have influenced how health is constructed and understood in society today. These are:

- shifts in meanings of health
- the use of telematics in health care
- health choices.

Shifts in meanings of health

During the latter half of this century, both public and professional views on health and health care have changed. There are a number of reasons for this. The universal adoption of biomedicine as the basis for health care throughout the first three-quarters of this century has meant that, by separating the body out into 'bits of bits' (biopathology), we have lost sight of the health and well-being of the whole person.

The twentieth century has been an age of science and, in particular, medical science. Whereas society turned in previous centuries to priests or gods for meaning and leadership, now they turn to doctors. In what Armstrong (1993) refers to as 'the triumph of truth', medical scientists can demonstrate the existence of diseases previously hidden within the human body. Ill health was once attributed to evil air (miasmas) or evil eyes (curses); now it is attributed to abnormal physiology (diseases). 'Normal' physiology thus becomes equated with health.

Disease protection used to involve the invocation of rituals with charms and prayers. The twentieth century equivalents are low cholesterol diets and running shoes. 'Look after your heart' is not a plea for tolerance and understanding in society, but an exhortation (and a responsibility) to individuals to maintain efficient cardiovascular functioning.

Verbraak (1992) describes how the artefacts of this philosophy influence mass consciousness:

'Healthy behaviour, within certain modish margins, is part of a culturally expected lifestyle . . . the weighing scales in railway stations, supermarkets or hotel lobbies are being replaced by instruments to measure your blood pressure or to establish your mental composure. Professional advertising campaigns focus on better lifestyles, newspapers and television have weekly contributions on health and society. Joggers colour the countryside and golf, tennis and surfing clubs prosper.'

Challenges to scientific reductionism

Modern medicine has evolved from the scientific reductionist paradigm that has dominated social life in Western societies throughout this century. The paradigm is characterized by use of the systems theory. This describes everything from the functioning of the human body to the economic function- ing of societies (eg free market or communist). Systems theories are intellec- tually elegant and persuasive, but by stripping away the wealth of detail that is inherent in context, they become merely academic.

Worldwide, dissatisfaction with scientific reductionism as the only ex- planation for individual and social functioning is growing. Ormerod (1994) argues in *The death of economics* that economics' core axioms do not and cannot correspond to any known reality; economists know this but close their eyes to it because their theories have intellectual appeal.

In all areas of social life, the reductionist paradigm is undergoing serious challenge. Not only is it demonstrably lacking in human values and qualities; it simply doesn't work. This is as true of the medical model on which health care has been based in the twentieth century, as it is of the dominant economics model. The massive financial and human investment that has been made in high technology medicine has, in the main, not paid off. The financial cost of increasingly sophisticated diagnostic and treatment techniques needs to be offset against the moral and social costs often involved for patients and others whose less glamorous needs (eg social support) go underfunded and unmet.

Technological advances in medical care and increased research into health service issues have contributed to a dramatic rise in expenditure on health care in Europe. Despite this, the health of the European people has not improved as much as might have been expected. The problems caused by chronic diseases, disabilities, new epidemics such as AIDS and illicit drug consumption are increasingly worrying, not only to governments, but also to individuals. At the same time, there are serious concerns about the efficacy of sophisticated technology and existing health services that rely heavily on hospital and specialized medicine to confront those problems (Dutton, 1988; Konner, 1993).

Health For All: ideology and targets

Pressures from rising demand for health care in Europe (reflected in increased expenditure) have forced many countries to examine a range of options for changing the system. This is a common problem in spite of differences between individual health care systems. A potential solution is the develop- ment of a better system of primary health care with an emphasis on the twin goals of cost efficiency and service effectiveness. A number of strategies are being pursued by European Union (EU) countries to achieve these objectives. The common factor linking such efforts is the Health For All (HFA) ideology propounded by the World Health Organization (WHO, 1978 and subsequent). HFA is based on the use of a social, rather than a medical, model of health.

In 1978, WHO issued the Alma Ata Declaration. This recognized Health For All as a fundamental right and saw reorientation of resources towards primary health care as the way to achieve it. In 1985, 38 targets for HFA were set for countries in the WHO European Region (revised 1992). The European governments that were signatory to the 1985 agreement have in principle accepted the obligation to work on health targets.

There are three groups of targets. The first is aimed at reducing inequalities between countries and social groups. The inequalities identified are concerned with traditional preventive care (eg reducing maternal and infant mortality) and new public health issues, such as reducing traffic accidents and deaths by suicide.

The second set of targets addresses changes in lifestyle, the environment and provision of health care. The scope of this group is vast, covering policy and structural changes necessary for the adoption of healthy lifestyles, promotion of positive health behaviour, and action on air pollution, hazardous waste, water pollution and food contamination. Also advocated are healthy homes, schools and workplaces and a redistribution of resources from secondary to primary care.

The third set of targets identifies the necessary support frameworks as research, information systems, policy and planning frameworks and the education and training of health and other public service workers.

A major vehicle for putting these targets into operation is the Healthy Cities movement, in which the principles of partnership, team-work and collaboration are employed in planning for health (see Ashton, 1992). Healthy Cities philosophy is underpinned by principles contained in the 1986 Ottawa Charter. In this, the need for reorientation of health services to primary health care is addressed, as are the needs to strengthen community action, create supportive environments, develop personal skills and build a healthy public policy.

The HFA philosophy places more emphasis on health promotion than on treatment and care. Key features are:

- community responsiveness and representation

- collaboration and partnership in service planning, delivery and evaluation

- multidisciplinary teamworking (professional, voluntary and lay)

- equity in service distribution

- measures to redress health inequalities (ie social justice in care access and provision)

- individual and community development.

Health promotion: medical and social models

The social model of health is concerned with the conditions and contexts that shape health opportunities and illness experiences. Recognition of the value of the social model of health has been responsible for the development of a new health paradigm: health promotion. The emerging discipline of health promotion encompasses three strands:

- preventive care
- health education
- health protection.

Preventive care involves screening and diagnostic activities (medical model), and also social interventions such as immunization against specific diseases. A sensitive community diagnosis indicates appropriate interventions (social model). **Health education** may be individualistic and disease focused (medical model), or collective and health oriented (social model). **Health protection** is concerned with both remedial and rehabilitative care (medical model), and promotion of full health potential (social model).

Generally, medical models are reactive whilst social models are proactive. There is a need for both types of model and both sets of action. The social model is longer term, visionary and encompasses all citizens, whilst the medical model is more immediate, more narrowly focused and relates to significantly fewer individuals. The medical model can quite comfortably be accommodated within a social model of health; indeed this is the case made in *The New Public Health* (Ashton and Seymour, 1988). Too frequently, however, the medical model is chosen as the sole vehicle for policy making. *The New Public Health* has its origins in the WHO HFA movement. It recognizes the need for a range of strategies to be employed in health care delivery and health promotion and acknowledges that society needs to care for those already ill, as well as promote the health and interests of those who are not ill, but may be vulnerable.

Conflicting models of health operate in society and produce inequalities in health experiences and opportunities. Medical reductionism causes fragmentation of social policy and champions particular policy approaches over others. The social backdrop of scientific reductionism that has influenced policy making in this century has led policy makers to base decisions on medical models. However, health practitioners who have adopted HFA values are not comfortable when forced to act exclusively within the confines of the medical model; doing so provokes extreme role conflict.

Gott and O'Brien (1990) have explored the role of the nurse in health promotion. They identified how nurses are required to work to a medical model of health to carry out their nursing tasks (giving health advice), yet their personal and professional values are rooted in a social model:

> 'Today it's the "in thing" to go jogging, to be "green", to be "ozone friendly" and I don't think that's such an issue for someone lower down the social scale. I think they're more interested in scraping a living together and their day to day existence . . . I think we don't give a very good deal to those who most need the services because they end up with the middle-class body governing their lives.' (*health visitor*)

Jonkers-Kuiper (1992) describes the conflicting health models and agendas surrounding implementation of the Collective Prevention Health Care Act in The Netherlands and notes similar problems to those described above. Other authors (Siler-Wells, 1988; Jacobson *et al.*, 1991) challenge the Western policy focus on individualistic (medical model) 'risk reducing' interventions (eg screening) at the expense of health promoting (community-wide) interventions. They comment that lifestyle (and victims) are socially constructed.

A 'risk reduction' approach is appropriate for disease prevention. However health and well-being demand a broader approach encompassing the promotion of quality of everyday life in homes and communities. With regard to sustained behaviour change, a community development approach offers the greatest chance of success (Beattie, 1988; Lefebvre, 1991). Moreover, interventions alone are insufficient to protect and promote health. There needs to be a supportive framework of healthy public policies and an understanding and commitment by health professionals (service providers) to work together.

Several authors (Jones, 1990; Gott and O'Brien, 1990; Godinho *et al.*, 1992) have noted the imperative for health professionals to change from paternalistic to co-operative practices. There are marked differences, however, in views of how this should be done. Some see the changed role for health professionals as simply giving more and 'better' information:

> 'The professionals will need better teaching, counselling and decision-making skills to communicate with patients and help them in their decision-making . . . people will continue to be afraid, worried or imagining illnesses, but relevant multimedia presentation can make the best use of specialist skills and disseminate the material widely. Not all patients will be able to participate in this way, but facilities should be developed to allow the majority to participate at the level that they can accept and understand.' (Roger France and Santucci, 1991)

Others (Beattie *et al.*, 1993) call for 'bottom up' citizens' initiatives to promote health. (Examples of 'good practice' in co-operative working can be found in Health For All initiatives such as the Health Cities movement (Ashton, 1992) and the European Community's Tipping The Balance (TTB) Project (Godinho *et al.*, 1992)).

Tipping The Balance

The approach of TTB (research based on case studies of good practice) has been legitimized as a European priority action area (*see* Leadbetter, 1992, *European health services handbook*):

> 'In many fields, but perhaps particularly public health, there is felt to be a need for models of innovative good practice . . . The following action programmes could be envisaged:
>
> - health service programmes emphasizing the important role of primary health care (PHC)
>
> - action on health inequalities.'

The TTB seven country European Community action research project focused on shifting the philosophical, funding and organizational balance towards PHC by readdressing the ratio of PHC to (disproportionate) secondary health care activity. The operational definition of PHC which was used reflects the spirit of Health For All. Four ways of interpreting PHC were identified:

- as a philosophy, reinforcing notions of justice and equity

- as a principle, incorporating the notion of free, open, and relevant access to all who need it

- as the first point of health care contact

- as a set of activities concerned with disease prevention and treatment, rehabilitation and health promotion.

The philosophies underpinning the TTB project (equity, PHC and the value of case study research) helped shape the direction of this project on telehealth and telemedicine.

Input from technologists

Technologists are also service providers. Comparatively little is published on the role of technologists in telemedicine (Jones, 1990), but there are lots of exhortations for technologists to work more closely with users (*see*, in particular, Biag, 1991). Dalton (1986) gives evidence that this may already be happening:

> 'Research groups in both Germany and the UK investigated fetal phono-cardiology. Each of the groups had strong bio-engineering support, and it

was the engineers who showed how sophisticated techniques . . . might be applied to fetal heart sounds to reveal useful information. Their short-term goal was simply to improve fetal data collection, but in the longer term they foresaw a better understanding of fetal physiology, and thereby an improvement in fetal health and well-being.'

The use of telematics in health care

The transmission of information across distances (telematics) is rapidly increasing within the EU. This is hardly surprising, as it reflects a worldwide trend with which the EU, as a major economic force, needs to keep pace. Current EU research policy (Fourth Framework Programme/Research and Technological Development 1994–98) is as follows:

'The research in the field of telematic applications in areas of common interest will have two aims. One will be to promote the competitiveness of European industry . . . the other . . . is to promote research activities necessary for other common policies.'

Telematics in medicine has been largely concerned with data handling (eg relating to medical records), drug prescribing and surveillance. Computerization of patient and client primary health care records is now routine in the northern European countries and is set to become standard throughout Europe.

Diagnostic screening

Increasingly, telematics is used for screening activities. Screening is made possible because of increasingly sophisticated diagnostic technologies. Screening for (existing) disease is the major PHC growth activity in Europe. Given that coronary heart disease, strokes and cancers are the major killer diseases in Europe (around 70% all deaths, combined), it is unsurprising that efforts should be made to identify and treat those at risk. However, there are problems with screening:

- Little policy or budgetary attention is paid to preventing people getting the diseases in the first place (eg healthy home/workplace and nutrition policies).

- Once a disease is established, screening is only marginally useful.

- Screening tests are often highly inaccurate, particularly the cervical screening programme which errs heavily on the side of false positives, needlessly scaring vast numbers of women every year.

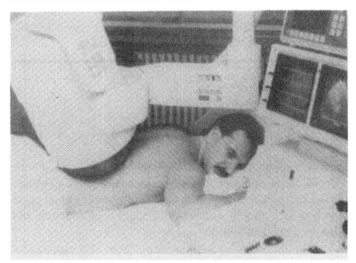

Figure 1:   A man undergoing a diagnostic scan

Ebeling and Nischan (1992) report a screening programme to control lung cancer in Germany by analysing data using two case control studies. Mortality from lung cancer did not appear to be affected by the screening programmes studied. They found that the high cost of mass screening, combined with uncertainty about the benefits of early treatment of lung cancer, outweigh any advantages of such screening. This finding is in line with the view of D'Souza (1992) who argues for the need to redirect spending to prevention of medical conditions, rather than simply labelling them as he claims screening does.

Telemedicine

In addition to the use of telematics in record handling and screening/diagnosis, remote telematic 'care' (telemedicine) is also enjoying rapid growth. Telemedicine has been defined as 'the investigation, monitoring and management of patients, and the education of patients and staff using systems which allow ready access to expert advice, no matter where the patient is located' (Van Goor and Christensen, 1992). On the use of telemedicine, Venters (1990) notes:

'Telemedicine allows the *in vivo* monitoring of patients which enables the accurate definition of the clinical status of the patient and assessment of the impact of therapies on the outcomes for the patient. As a result of such an assessment, informed choices can be made on appropriate treatment both for the individual patients and specific groups with a particular condition.'

Currently the major effort in telemedicine is in diagnosis and monitoring physiological dysfunction. In medicine itself, however, there has been a resurgence of interest in holism (Pietroni, 1993) with the realization that physiology is only part of what makes a person, and a refocusing on health promotion as opposed to illness care. In the sphere of telematics, this allows for a holist rather than a reductionist view of health which includes, but is not exclusively, telemedicine. There is a place for telemedicine in health care, but not the hegemonically dominant place it now occupies.

Telehealth

Telemedicine is reductionist. Telehealth, on the other hand, offers enormous potential for health promotion and illness prevention. Telehealth has been defined as (Veneris, 1992):

> 'The provision of telematic services and related goods which can provide telemedicine services and assist in raising the consciousness and increasing the involvement of both the individual and the community towards the total health environment . . . aiming to improve well-being and wellness.'

The definition of telehealth that has emerged during this study, and is preferred, is 'The promotion and facilitation of health and well-being with individuals and communities, by use of telematic services'.

Social technologies

According to Milio (1992), technology is neutral; it can be used for the benefit of mankind, or misused. However, like the nuclear bomb, it can't be uninvented! The existence of technology, particularly in the hands of powerful people (policy makers, doctors and other 'gate keepers') is a source of concern for some (Hancock, 1992):

> 'The information society can be a threat to our physical, mental and social well-being and we should learn to recognize it and treat it as a threat. That way, we might at least reduce the health effect somewhat, and learn at the same time how to enhance the potential health benefits.'

Technology, therefore, may be seen as a threat to personal freedoms and opportunities; investing in technology reflects and reinforces the dominant cultural ideology and can put powerful tools in the hands of powerful people.

Whilst the discussion so far has focused on medical technologies, social technologies are also relevant; indeed they may have a greater role to play in health promotion and illness prevention than medical technologies. Social technologies include 'everyday' things such as the television and the telephone. In order to satisfy mass market demands for effectiveness and efficiency, they need to be 'user friendly'. They are also, generally, low technology. Study of these services was therefore considered particularly appropriate.

Social interaction and integration also merit consideration. The popular view is that use of technology reduces social interaction: Stuurop (1992) cites the French philosopher Jean Baudrillard (1986, *Amerique*):

'It is a culture that thinks up both special institutions in which bodies can touch one another, and frying pans in which water doesn't touch the bottom of the pan . . . That is what they call interface or interaction. This had replaced the face to face contact and the action, and that is now what they call communication. . . . That is what now constitutes information, and it has trickled through like a phobic and manic underlying principle that affects erotic relations as much as it affects kitchen utensils.'

Social interaction is a normal and necessary feature of living and participating in a society, thus feeling a valued and worthwhile member of it. Some social groups, owing to age, disease or disability, experience less social contacts and consequently are less socially integrated than others. Indeed it has been noted (Gott and Packham, 1993) that some housebound people, particularly the elderly, value the social contact function of health care provision (home nursing) as highly as the service itself.

One application of telemedicine is remote home care. It is possible that remote home care could reduce the number of visits health workers make to people's homes, potentially compounding social isolation for an already disadvantaged group. Social integration has therefore been identified as an important variable for investigation.

Health choices

Europe comprises rich and poor countries. Each has different priorities and budgets for health care. Additionally, technologies vary, as do the decisions made about their value and use. This predisposes to inequalities because of unequal budget allocations for high technology versus preventive care, and limited access to high technology care. On equality of access to information, Veneris (1992) notes, 'health care poor areas are most often also information network poor'.

The EU countries are moving towards market-driven cost containment in health care. Open-ended health budgets will no longer exist so health choices will have to be made. A national debate, Choices in Health Care, began in 1992 in The Netherlands (*see* the report published by the Government Committee on Choices in Health Care in 1992) with the intention of promoting public discussion of issues concerning choice and public responsibility in health care. The report addresses issues relevant to all EU countries, indeed all Western countries, and is principally concerned with 'value for money' in health care. Similar discussions have been going on in both the UK and Germany.

There are a variety of ways of funding service provision. In all European countries there is a mix of public and private provision (to a differing degree). Hutton (1991) has usefully distinguished between two systems:

1 **Public health care systems**. These are owned, planned, managed and financed by public authorities. Examples of such systems are in the UK, Denmark, Ireland and Italy.

2 **Social security health care systems**. These are planned by public authorities but funded by insurance agencies belonging to the social security system. Health care is provided by institutions in public and private ownership. Examples exist in France, Germany, Greece, The Netherlands, Portugal and Spain.

Social trends in Europe indicate the likelihood of decreased collective taxation, so choices will have to be made about which services and products are most needed, and are socially and economically 'worth' providing. This raises issues such as prioritization and the rationing of services and products, and the need to control and evaluate innovations more carefully. Whatever socioeconomic solutions are chosen, reorientation of service provision towards primary health care is likely to occur.

Primary health care systems

In comparison to the hospital sector, the primary health care (prevention) sector has been grossly underfunded (Godinho *et al.*, 1991). In Europe, the proportion of spending on primary care (as opposed to hospital care) varies markedly. It is around 10% in the UK, as opposed to 40% in Finland. There has, of late, been increased recognition in all the EU countries that to provide effective and efficient health care for European citizens, a greater percentage of the health budget needs to be re-allocated to primary health care.

Primary health care systems are, in general, fairly extensively developed in the northern European countries, and less developed in southern European countries. With regard to service organization, WHO (1986) has noted:

'In some countries, well co-ordinated teams form the established and recognized first point of contact with the official health system. In others, access to (primary) health care may be through general practitioners, specialists or nurses, each working alone.'

In addition to differences in service organization, there may also be differences in orientation. A distinction needs to be made between primary health care services and primary medical services. Primary health care services are characterized by integration of medical care with social, educational and other proactive health services, and draw on a social model of health. Primary medical services are characterized by reactive, individualistic and preventive treatment and care activities, and draw on a medical model of health. The distinction is important because, owing to the escalation of medical costs throughout Europe, some governments are currently exploring ways of reducing costs by promoting certain forms of provision (individualistic screening and health education), and reducing other forms (community development and collaboration).

The myopic and misguided reductionist trend that has dominated health policy for most of this century seems in danger of being perpetuated. Yet reorientation to primary health care, together with sensitive and sensible use of telematic support services, offers a new and potentially more effective direction for health care in the twenty-first century. This has been recognized by the EU in its Framework for Action in the Field of Public Health programme (CEC [1993] 559). This sets out the Commission's proposals for taking forward the European Community's work on public health to meet the objective introduced by the Treaty on European Union that 'the Community shall contribute towards ensuring a high level of human health protection'.

The approach will include the establishment of common objectives and networks, exchange of information and personnel, improvement of data systems, financial support to programmes and projects, production of an annual Community health report, and assistance to cost reduction efforts.

Summary

The model of health care that has dominated the twentieth century is a model of illness: the medical model. It is reductionist in its focus in that it is primarily concerned with (bits of) individual physiological functioning. There has been increasing dissatisfaction with the model and its dominance. It is neither socially nor economically effective. Policy-makers are now moving towards adoption of a different model of health: the social model.

The social model of health has its origins in the World Health Organization's Health For All movement. It recognizes the interrelated influences of social, political and economic factors on health opportunities and illness experiences.

Despite this, current health policy is characterized by continuing use of the medical model and in particular the 'risk reduction' approach. Such an approach is appropriate for disease prevention, but health and well-being rely on the promotion of quality of everyday life in homes and communities. Primary, rather than secondary, care is necessary to help deliver this.

The use of telematics in medicine is increasing. To date, telemedicine has consumed a vast amount of resources and delivered much data, but little in the way of improvement in quality of life (Tetzchner, 1991; Humphreys, 1992). Telemedicine technologies are limited in their scope. As far as health promotion is concerned, the social technologies (telephones, televisions, etc) are also relevant; indeed they may have a greater role to play in health promotion and illness prevention than the medical technologies. The potential for telehealth by use of social technologies is therefore a central feature of this study.

2 Telehealth and Telemedicine: A Case Study Approach

'... there is a need for models of innovative good practice ...'

(European health services handbook, 1992)

The aim of this book is to find and describe 'good practice' in the promotion of health and well-being by use of telematic services. Health promotion is deemed the facilitation of positive health and the prevention of ill health. It involves health education, disease prevention (screening and surveillance) and health protection (healthy public policies).

The research goals were:

- to find and describe a set of 'good practice' case studies

- to analyse the social impact of these case studies

- to consider the policy options raised by the case studies.

The baseline methodology involved literature review and discussions with experts. Previous work commissioned by the European Foundation (Veneris, 1992) on the social impact of telemedicine at home proved to be a valuable source document, particularly with regard to technical information.

In addition to literature review, Delphic-type discussions with experts were held to identify further and review key research concepts and issues. Using networks already known to the author and her advisers, new networks were discovered and accessed. As a result of this communications occurred with key people in a number of European and North American Institutions and countries. A combination of postal, telephone, facsimile and face-to-face communications took place. In all, around 140 people and 45 Institutions were contacted, representing 14 different developed countries. Meetings with the Research Manager, other officials and other researchers from the European Foundation, and with European Community officials in Brussels were particularly helpful.

Future researchers and others who need to understand in detail how the European Community/Union developed, and how it works, are referred to an excellent handbook, published in 1993 and edited by Neil Leadbetter, the *European health services handbook*. For those who just need a brief guide, the following summary should suffice.

The European Union

The EU is served by a single institutional framework which respects the national identity of its member states. Of particular interest in the field of health care, the Treaty on European Union calls upon the activities of the EU to be widened to include health protection. On 1st January 1993, the 12 member states of the EU became a single economic entity with a combined population of 342 million people – approximately 6.4% of the world population.

The European Commission is the policy planning body responsible for the administration of the Union and its funds. It proposes Union legislation and executes decisions taken by the Council of Ministers.

The Council of Ministers is responsible for passing Community law, on the basis of policy proposals put forward by the Commission, and following consultation with the directly elected members of the European Parliament. The Government of each of the 12 member states is represented on the Council. In most cases, decisions are taken on the basis of a majority rule.

The European Parliament is made up of 567 members (MEPs), directly elected by the citizens of the 12 member states for a five-year term of office. When a proposal is submitted to the Parliament, it is considered by one or more of its 20 permanent committees, one of which is the Committee on the Environment, Public Health and Consumer Protection. With 44 members, this is one of the largest of the European Parliament's permanent committees. The membership is broadly representative of the strengths of the political groups in the Parliament and all nine languages of the Union are normally represented.

Executive functions are carried out by 22 Directorates–General (DGs), based in Brussels and Luxembourg (*see* Figure 2).

The EU's research policy aims to complement national research efforts through the commissioning of projects which can more effectively be carried out at a European, as opposed to national, level. Framework programmes have been used since the mid 1980s to announce strategic objectives and to indicate the amounts of money available for their realization. Continuity between Framework programmes (ie the Third and Fourth) is maintained by continuing high levels of expenditure on such areas as information technology, telecommunications, and industrial and materials technologies. Together, these account for more than half of the total research budget.

The European Commission is the executive arm of the Union; its task is to propose measures based on articles from the founding treaties and to ensure that they are implemented. It is organized as follows:

DG I	External relations	DG XIII*	Telecommunications, information market and exploitation of research
DG II	Economic and financial affairs		
DG III*	Industry		
DG IV	Competition	DG XIV	Fisheries
DG V*	Employment, industrial relations and social affairs	DG XV	Internal market and financial services
DG VI*	Agriculture	DG XVI	Regional policies
DG VII	Transport	DG XVII	Energy
DG VIII	Development	DG XVIII	Credit and investments
DG IX	Personnel and administration	DG XIX	Budgets
DG X	Audiovisual media, information, communication and culture	DG XX	Financial control
		DG XXI	Customs and indirect taxation
DG XI*	Environment, nuclear safety and civil protection	DG XXIII	Enterprise policy, distributive trades, tourism and co-operatives
DG XII*	Science, research and development		

*Although no specific reference to health is made in the 1957 Treaty of Rome and there is no DG for health within the Commission, the starred DGs produce policy which has some impact on health, as follows: DG III – mutual recognition of diplomas, pharmaceuticals, food, medical equipment and standardization; DG V – health and safety, public health, Europe against cancer, Europe against AIDS, nutrition; DG VI – pesticides, veterinary medicine, nutrition; DG XI – radiation protection, environmental monitoring and inspection; DG XII – nuclear safety research, biotechnology, medical research; DG XIII – information technology, advanced informatics in medicine.

Figure 2: The European Commission

Health and technology Framework programmes

Research in all those DGs involved in health and technology matters was explored for potential case study material for this book. The programmes that yielded opportunities for inclusion were:

- DG XIII: AIM (now Telematics in Health Care), RACE, and TIDE

- DG V: HANDYNET/HELIOS.

Telematics in Health Care is by far the largest programme. The main area of activity is diagnosis and surveillance for clinical decision making. Projects of interest with regard to health promotion include fetal monitoring and diabetic self care.

RACE (Research and Development in Advanced Communications Technologies in Europe) (project R 1054) involves telephony services for people with special needs. Experiments are taking place in Germany, The Netherlands, Italy, Sweden, Finland and Portugal.

TIDE (Technology Initiative for Disabled and Elderly people) is a research and development initiative aimed at stimulating the creation of a single market in rehabilitation technology in Europe.

HANDYNET is part of the HELIOS (Handicapped People in the European Community Living in an Open Society) programme. HELIOS is in its second action phase and aims to achieve the social and economic integration of disabled people in the EU. HANDYNET is a telematic networking system for disabled people, their helpers, health professionals and policy makers.

Choice of method

The approach chosen for data collection and interpretation was a phenomenological one, involving both quantitative and qualitative work. This method was considered most appropriate to the exploration of a newly emerging and complex paradigm: telehealth.

When compared to methods generally used in traditional medical research, this approach may appear to be 'unscientific'. This is entirely deliberate. Feyerband (1975) challenges the 'scientific' approach as myopic and misfounded:

> 'Science is much closer to myth than a scientific philosophy is prepared to admit . . . (It is useful) . . . only for those who have already decided in favour of a certain ideology, or who have accepted it without having ever examined its advantages and its limits . . . It is thus possible to create a tradition that is held together by strict rules, and that is also successful to some extent. But is it desirable to support such a tradition to the exclusion of everything else? Should we transfer to it the sole rights for dealing in knowledge, so that any result that has been obtained by any other methods is at once ruled out of court? . . . My answer will be a resounding *no*.'

In making this point the intention is not to denigrate the role of medical research as such, rather to point out the need for all types of methodology, and to make space for all types of accounts of events. Reductionist medical research is entirely appropriate for studies of physiological functioning and malfunctioning. It is inappropriate for studying the human condition as a whole.

Support for this choice of methodology in an area of study such as the one selected also comes from Johnson (1990) and Broughton (1991), both of whom recommend use of a phenomenological approach when dealing with an area of complexity such as that represented by this study.

Choice of case studies

Choice of case studies was influenced by a belief in the validity of the Health For All criteria, set out in Chapter 1.

It emerged quite early in the life of the project that, with regard to telematics, Health For All is not currently being promoted very successfully. Impressions gained as a result of an extensive document review (AIM programme in particular), and discussions with experts were that:

- telemedicine work is primarily for the benefit of industry and service providers

- most goes on at the hospital to PHC interface

- the focus is mainly diagnosis, surveillance and information management

- patient involvement is largely directed at compliance

- while many publications advocate health education, health promotion and consumer involvement the rhetoric seems not to be reflected in practice

- health promotion seems to be interpreted as traditional preventive and health education activities, using the new technologies (ie providing more of the same, in a more spectacular manner).

AIM Research and Development Action Workplan 1991–94 (see CEC, 1993) does, however, report the shortage of services to the growing segments of primary and home care. Also reported is that the trend 'continues away from institutional treatment into home or ambulatory care', and that 'many groups would benefit (from telemedicine services) . . . including pregnant women, newborn and paediatric groups, adults at risk, the chronically ill and those with motor disability and age related pathologies'.

In preliminary discussions about the project, almost everyone made the point that the technological 'push' had come from above and consumers' views were rarely represented. This book argues that services to groups identified as being in need should be addressed, and that examples of 'good practice' in service provision should be identified and promoted. Conclusions reached about choice of case studies were therefore that:

- they should focus on the overall promotion of health and well-being

- they should be low to medium technology

- the results of the study should be applicable to poorer, as well as richer European countries.

There should be:

- a balance between health domains (populations and type of activity such as prevention and care, health education, health protection)

- a geographical balance in terms of countries selected

- research feasibility (resources versus constraints)

- potential for transfer of 'good practice'.

It was considered important that the sample population should reflect certain demographic and sociological characteristics. Thus the focus was on broad population groups and those with the opportunity to change. It was therefore considered important to study pregnant women, adolescents, disabled, and elderly people.

Case studies chosen were:

1 domiciliary fetal monitoring (DFM) (formerly an AIM project)

2 health education via a computer youth network (E ZOOT)

3 HELIOS/HANDYNET computer information system for the disabled

4 personal alarm systems for the elderly (TIDE project)

5 social support via videophones (RACE project)

6 public participation in decision making.

The samples

Each specific case study sample comprised interviews with all the key actors, consumers, providers, and institutional policy makers. A list of contacts for each case study area is shown in the Appendix. The samples comprised service providers and users situated in 15 locations in seven countries.

DFM (Wales) obstetricians, midwives and researchers were seen at their place of work and users were seen in their homes.
E ZOOT (Canada): providers were seen at their place of work and users were communicated with using the electronic Bulletin Board.

HANDYNET (The Netherlands and Italy): technologists, researchers and primary care staff were seen at their place of work, whilst users were seen at local centres and their homes.

Alarm systems (The Netherlands, Canada): engineers and service managers were seen in work settings; users were contacted by telephone and through home visits.

Videotelephony (Frankfurt, Portugal): engineers and service managers were seen at their place of work, whilst users were visited by videotelephone and in their own homes.

Public participation (Canada, USA) providers were seen at their place of work, users were reached electronically.

It had originally been planned to include another case study setting (Greece: alarm system), but following lengthy and complex negotiations this goal had to be abandoned.

Data collection and analysis

Data collection involved analysis of existing material available at each case study site and elsewhere, face-to-face interviews with key actors, and field observations of systems in use.

Prior to visiting a location personal contact was made with a key person by telephone. This initial contact was followed up with a letter or facsimile in the person's native language in order that the project could be both understood fully and explained to others.

A simple check-list was used to collect field data (*see* collapsed version in Figure 3). More sophisticated measures were considered inappropriate due to the differing purposes, natures and cultures surrounding each case study.

Observation data notes were designed to capture quality criteria as follows:

- technical aspects/fitness for purpose

- interface characteristics

- environmental ethos (*see* Donabedian, 1980, 1982 and 1985).

Technical aspects are concerned with fitness for purpose: does the service do what it is supposed to do; does it do it efficiently and effectively; is what is offered appropriate?

Interface characteristics are about how the service is delivered and perceived. Interpersonal relationships between providers and users are important, as is evidence of team working. Consumers need to have confidence that workers know what each other are doing and why: that there is a coherent, defensible, shared vision for service delivery.

Project: Location:

Key person: Technology:

Population served (age, sex, ethnicity, class):

Scale:

Resources funding:

Origination/recognition of need (when, why, who?):

How was support obtained?

What were the obstacles?

Management:

What factors helped implementation?

Who is involved in service planning, delivery, evaluation?

How is continuity/quality ensured?

Which other agencies collaborate/how?

How are citizens involved; how are their rights protected?

How is the service advertised?

What is the 'take up'/why/changed at all?

How were providers selected and trained?

The future:

What are the planned future developments?

What are the foreseen challenges?

What recommendations would be useful for similar services?

Figure 3:   The case study check-list

Environmental aspects are concerned with the physical and social ethos in which service delivery occurs and its conduciveness to participatory relationships between users and workers: is the service run for the benefit of the providers or the people, and is it run for all of the people or only some of them?

These criteria were specifically selected to relate to the HFA principles of service quality/effectiveness, teamwork/collaboration and user responsiveness.

All material was collected by the author. Following transcription of notes, audiotapes and other primary sources, full transcripts were sent to the initial contact, to check their accuracy and veracity. Participants proved to be extremely helpful and generous with their time and comments.

With regard to evaluation, the Memorial University Telemedicine Centre (MUTEC) has evolved eight guidelines for the introduction and evaluation of technological innovations. Their criteria (shown below) were also included:

- Use the simplest, least expensive technology that will meet needs.

- Develop a flexible system.

- Involve all user groups from the inception of the project.

- Seek the support of administrative personnel at health care sites.

- Plan carefully for the co-ordination of the system at all levels.

- Develop a consortium of users within and outside the health services.

- Plan for continuity of service beyond the demonstration period.

- Include evaluation.

Together, data sets were designed to yield the following information:

- type of innovation (technical, preventive care, health education/promotion, health protection)

- quality/success of technological innovation

- degree of client/community responsiveness achieved

- equity of service of product distribution

- degree of collaboration/teamwork amongst service providers

- consideration of ethical issues

- implications for change in service provision, policy, training and research.

Presenting the case studies

Each study deals with a different topic, a different population, a different set of issues, and a different set of 'key actors'. Everyone who participated was exceedingly generous with their time, resources and information; nevertheless some areas were more difficult to collect data in than others. Two major concerns for some participants were both confidentiality of data they already held, and the status of technical data, which they saw as being associated with the commercial viability of the product or innovation being investigated. This was particularly true of videotelephones. Ironically, the participants who guarded data most closely included some who were already involved in other EC projects.

For these reasons, directly comparable sets of data for all six case studies are not available for presentation. However, much common data exists and it has been possible to follow a common format in data presentation. All the major issues that the study sought to address are represented in the data.

Presentation of the case studies includes:

- reviews and presentations of associated published and 'in house' literature
- field observations on visits to service institutions and people's homes
- excerpts of field interviews, made during visits to case study locations.

Presentation follows a common format using the following headings:

- type of service
- technology
- location
- population
- context (including programme origins and local demography)
- technical description (including costs where available)
- service description (including quality aspects, teamwork and user responsiveness)
- users (including users' experiences, views and evaluations)

- future plans (including planned developments and obstacles)

- review (each individual case study visit is followed by brief observational comments on both social impact and relevant policy issues. Each chapter concludes with a summary).

Full analysis and discussion of case studies occurs in Chapter 9. A glossary of abbreviations of technical organizations and terms is provided at the end of the book.

Summary

The aim of the research was to find, analyse and disseminate good practice in use of telematics to promote health (telehealth). The method chosen to do this was by selection of case studies. Case studies were drawn from existing EC research programmes, and also from Canada and the USA. Very broad study populations were selected in order that the potential for transfer of good practice could be fully realized. Some standard criteria were elucidated to aid presentation of case studies.

3 Telehealth and Pregnant Women

'It depends whether you view pregnancy as an illness or a normal process.'

(service provider)

Type of service

Domiciliary fetal monitoring (DFM), to monitor fetuses identified as 'at risk' (formerly an AIM programme).

Technology

Remote monitoring using transfer of digital signals by Modem device. Monitors are used by pregnant women, in their own homes, and signals are transmitted to an obstetric unit for interpretation using the public telephone network system. Reduced data (from 20–30 minutes of continuous monitoring) are transmitted in less than 40 seconds.

DFM needs to be distinguished from the continuous electrical fetal monitoring (EFM) that is (often inappropriately) routinely applied to women during labour. The routine monitoring of all women during labour has been severely criticized in the 1992 Winterton Report. DFM is a totally different application which allows for early intervention in high risk pregnancies. Continuous EFM of an otherwise normal woman in the context of a hospital setting tethers the woman to the bed at the time of labour, hooks her up with equipment and causes the focus of care to shift from the woman to a machine. As will be seen with DFM, its application, and the relationship engendered with the patient are very different.

Location

Two settings in Wales; one urban (Cardiff), the other remote rural (the Valleys).

Population

'High risk' pregnant women.

Context

The Welsh DFM project was formerly an AIM Demonstration Pilot (1988–90). Antenatal Care Demonstrator projects are described by Dripps *et al.* (1992) in the IOS publication *Advances in medical informatics.*

All antenatal care services in the UK are offered free to all citizens, according to need. DFM is therefore available to anyone judged to be in need. A preliminary randomized study of DFM carried out in Cardiff (Dawson *et al.*, 1988; Middlemiss *et al.*, 1989) showed:

- reductions of time spent in hospital amongst this population of high risk mothers
- lower anxiety levels in high risk women monitored at home
- maternal satisfaction with the service provided.

Following successful implementation of DFM in an urban setting (Cardiff) the research team decided to investigate its potential with a rural population. (The Home Antenatal Care in the Valleys Project; 1990–94). This project was funded by the Valleys Initiative Programme of the Welsh Office. Its aim was to evaluate clinical, social and economic factors in the provision of domiciliary care for women with identified high risk pregnancies. At the time of data collection two locations were being studied, both in the South Wales Valleys, serving largely rural, scattered populations.

A multidisciplinary team designed, and is administering, the project. It is exploring:

- maternal satisfaction with the maternity care offered (longitudinal study)
- the social , clinical and economic benefits of a domiciliary antenatal care scheme run by community midwives for women with an identified high risk pregnancy (randomized study).

The (high) risk status of women is decided by the obstetrician, with regard to the following recognized risk factors:

- poor obstetric history (eg stillbirth or neonatal death)
- hypertension
- weight loss
- small for dates fetus
- diminished fetal movements
- minor antepartum haemorrhage.

The population being studied is quite deprived. A good flavour of population characteristics was provided at interview by the economist who is advising the project:

'Socially and economically it's a very depressed area . . . apart from Northern Ireland we're the most depressed on any of the indicators you care to mention . . . proportion of houses with indoor toilets . . . you're at the bottom of the league here. The main economic activity was coal mining, which has gone. (But) . . . community spirit is very strong here . . . you're much more likely to know your neighbours. When we first moved here, every half hour there was a knock on the door . . . they virtually organized a welcoming committee for us . . . being a deprived area there're lots of unmarried mothers and often not even a boyfriend on the scene . . . but Mum is there and Granny is there, it's different to big cities.'

As might have been expected, the economist had a good knowledge of, and strong views about the costs of everyday living. Regarding telephone ownership, he believed it to be:

'probably considerably less than the national average. It's something of a problem for home fetal monitoring . . . the midwife often has to go and find a phone.'

Access to an electricity supply is also sometimes a problem:

'The rate of disconnections has gone down so the statistics for the Electricity Board look good, but the reason for this is that if you are in arrears with your electricity bill they put you on a coin meter. If you don't have any money to put in the meter you don't have electricity . . . some of the midwives couldn't do traces because there was no money to feed the meter'.

With regard to official statistics, he cautioned that statistics like car ownership would be deceptive if applied to this population. The cars that *are* owned are invariably old and unreliable:

> 'The geography here is very unusual, towns run in ribbons along valleys . . . everyone's spread out, this causes enormous transport problems. Since the "free for all" with privatization of the buses, the transport system has declined drastically . . . there's an imperative to buy cars; there's more than average car ownership . . . that's an incredible amount of old bangers on the road.'

An ongoing trial of economic and social costs (Home Antenatal Care in the Valleys project) is being carried out. Patients are being requested to complete a weekly questionnaire and the results are expected during 1994.

Technical description

Monitors derive the fetal heart rate (FHR) from the Doppler shift wave form, produced by fetal heart movements when isolated by ultrasound from an external transducer on the mother's abdomen. A graphic record of FHR is produced on a printed strip. Some monitors also simultaneously record uterine activity using a simple transducer; all register fetal events such as movements. Newer monitors have a microprocessor which autocorrelates the returning signal, so averaging out the 'noise' made by other signals. This allows for a good quality signal to be received.

The senior research midwife described the scheme:

> 'Our area of working is women who need fetal heart monitoring or blood pressure monitoring who could be at home; in other words it's just purely the monitoring really that would be keeping them in hospital . . . they're actually doing a fetal heart trace of half an hour . . . the frequency depends on the reason why they need to have the monitoring in the first place, and they may be monitoring their own blood pressures as well and charting them and phoning them in.'

Around 70% of homes in Cardiff have telephones – ownership is lower in the Valleys. Even in the urban area, however, telephone ownership can be a problem:

> 'British Telecom just won't install phones in some Council housing estates. They say that the £200 installation costs and the rental won't be paid. Social security won't pay either. The point is that these women only need DFM for around three months, so the cost is negligible compared to in-patient care.' (research midwife)

Costs

Telephone call costs are borne by the user. Altogether (in Cardiff and the Valleys) there are 24 DFM machines. Machines currently cost around £7800 each. The service is not yet advertised as it is currently part of a research study. The envisaged need, however, is said to be not much greater than that currently available, as the vast majority of women enjoy uncomplicated pregnancies. Costs for the duration of the Home Antenatal Care in the Valleys Project are being met by the Valleys Initiative Programme of the Welsh Office. 'Hidden' costs are largely for extra staffing when existing staff are required to take on extra duties.

Service description

Services are based in the obstetric departments of a large urban teaching hospital (Cardiff), and a medium-sized rural hospital in a small town in the Valleys (Abergavenny).

There are some differences with regard to provision between Cardiff and the Valleys. In Cardiff domiciliary fetal monitoring is provided as part of an integrated package of antenatal care delivered by midwives working in close collaboration with consultant obstetricians:

'Once the consultant has assessed and feels, well, do they really need to be in hospital or can we monitor them at home, then if they can be monitored at home they are referred to me. I go out and see to the monitoring side but I do also urge them to go to mothercraft classes because I feel they need that social connection as well. They need to get to know the other mums, not just learn about pregnancy.' (research midwife)

Commenting on the fact that not all obstetricians favour DFM, the midwife went on to say:

'dealing with women who have lost babies before . . . every pregnancy is precious . . . some consultants say . . . all this monitoring . . . we don't need this . . . and yet when women are brought into hospital they don't seem to think about that . . . we are trying to give surveillance . . . and keep the monitoring as low as we can, but still be safe.'

The DFM scheme is part of the Cardiff Integrated Antenatal Care Scheme (CIACS). This offers home centred care for selected women with a high risk pregnancy. The intention is to provide continuity of care by making better use of midwifery and obstetric resources and to provide a new type of care (home based) when close surveillance is required.

According to the research obstetrician:

'DFM is only part of the package; the midwife is the central person, not the technology . . . but the technology has been the key that has unlocked the door . . . we're not promoting the technology, we're promoting the system that uses the technology.'

In Cardiff women are taught how to use DFM by one of the two research midwives. They phone the midwife at the receiving centre at a prearranged time, send their trace, and can talk with her if they wish to. Current evidence is that the women and the midwives are equally proficient at using the system:

'It keeps women at home. That's where they want to be and it's the best place for them. All they need is reassurance, and they can get that by monitoring themselves . . . and they're actually very good at it. They get very good tracings and keep their records well . . . in fact they put the hospital to shame; their records are better than ours many times!' (research midwife)

DFM was seen as appropriate for all social classes of high risk women:

'Women that have problems socially seem to do quite well on DFM say if they've been discharged from hospital, they get home and the attitude of their husband or partner is . . . well if you're home you must be OK . . . but once they have the machine the men take an interest in the technical side of it and also seem to give a little bit more attention to their partner because of it . . . they see that things can't all be straightforward if they've got a machine at home. Therefore I feel that these people are getting a little bit more attention and a little bit more rest and neighbours might be more willing to have the children . . . or take the children to school . . . so it gives them a little bit more clout . . . instead of just saying, "I have to rest," she can say, "Well, I've got this machine because baby's not growing so well" . . . so it works very well that way.' (research midwife)

In the Valleys, DFM is usually carried out by community midwives as part of their normal caseload. On some occasions patients monitor themselves. There are insufficient machines for each patient to keep one in their own home. Traces are sent into the obstetric unit at the local hospital. A computer programme has been designed to respond to abnormal traces and alert the obstetrician. Appropriate action can then be taken by the obstetric team.

According to the obstetrician, DFM is an ideal solution to meeting the needs of this type of deprived population:

'I think we've got eight out of the 10 socially deprived areas in Gwent (Region) in our catchment area, so we've got areas of great deprivation, very little money and they're stuck out in the back of beyond. There's high unemployment and high teenage pregnancy; we've got an illegitimacy rate of about 30%. One of the reasons we started DFM was that the buses are infrequent (when they run at all!) . . . Mrs Jones from Tredegar may spend an hour on the bus getting here and she may spend half an hour getting to the bus, she may be here by 11am; we may see her very promptly, but the next bus back is 2pm so she needs lunch out, which she can't afford, and she's back home at 3.30pm and there's another kid waiting outside the school at this time. Impossible. So just to attend a clinic is a day trip and if she has a family it's very, very expensive.'

Like the economist interviewed earlier, clinical staff in the Valleys also highlighted the problem of telephone ownership:

'I would suspect public phones are at a considerable distance from where they live, and a lot of them do get vandalized; I would not be happy thinking about a pregnant woman walking some distance from the house, particularly in the dark or bad weather. Also the cost of using the phone would have to be found.' (Valleys midwife)

This midwife went on to describe the problems faced by one user:

'It's a big, old, council estate up on the mountainside, very cold, and with lots of social problems. Anyway, when we pointed out that it would be difficult to get to (the user) every day, they decided that they could learn how to do it themselves. The midwife spent quite a long time with her and her husband and eventually they got it, and they can do it, apparently, quite well. A problem arose because there's no phone in the house, so the husband then went running around to the neighbours; he didn't know anybody with a phone but he went round asking and found someone about six doors down, and they allow him to transmit it (the trace) through, and he pays them a small sum. The arrangement is that she monitors herself in the morning but it's not transmitted till after midday, to get cheaper phone rates. So that was quite a problem really.

The other problem we ran into a few weeks ago was that the DFM machine we were (then) using wasn't battery operated, so it was run on the mains and the midwife started the monitor and the electricity went. The woman she was monitoring was on a token meter, and the minimum token value is £5. If you use up all your (tokens' worth) electricity you have a red button you press and you've got £5 worth emergency supply, but she'd already used that so all the supply had gone. So there they were, with no electricity at all and no money, so they had to wait until they could find a relative who could find the money to go down to town to buy the token (they needed £10 to get supply back) . . . so that was a little hiccup on that day.

DFM is more use to us for obstetric reasons in areas where there are lots of deprivation and social problems, but then, unfortunately, they are the ones that don't have a phone and this is the major handicap for us. This takes up a lot of midwife time . . . they spend a lot of time running back and forth helping them.'

Users

The five patients visited for this study represented the various types of user: married and unmarried, in private accommodation and council houses, teenagers through to mothers in their late thirties. One was being monitored during her first pregnancy following in-vitro fertilization; the others had poor obstetrics histories. DFM provides reassurance that the fetus is progressing normally.

The mothers had strong views about the need for midwifery support, and for staying at home:

'(the best thing is) having it there, I can listen to the baby's heartbeat anytime I want to.'
'It keeps me from getting worked up: it's there all the time in case I'm worried.'

This need for reassurance, and the effect a calm pregnancy could have on outcome was recognized by a research midwife the researcher spoke to – see page 36. Of course, if mothers have difficulty getting a signal, they become anxious:

'You can get frightened when you can't find the heart . . . it takes a long time sometimes.'

However, the midwife can point out (at a visit or by telephone) that, even with traditional methods and midwifery expertise, it is sometimes difficult to locate the fetal heart, particularly in the mid-months of pregnancy when the fetus is most mobile.

The researcher explored this area:

Researcher: 'Not everybody is really comfortable with machines and things like that. How did you feel when it was first suggested to you?'

User: 'All right, because with my job I worked with computers a lot like that, so, you know . . . I know what you mean . . . some people . . . like . . . well, my sister thought she'd be . . . you know . . . what will I do, I haven't got a clue, I don't know where all these leads go and all that, but I was all right. I took to it straightaway . . . I didn't find it difficult at all. It was easier than I thought it would be actually. I thought it would be . . .

you know . . . a bit more complicated, trying to find the heartbeat and everything, but it was great, it was good.'

Researcher: 'Can you remember what you felt like the first time you found it?'

User: 'Pleased (laughs) . . . it was funny because when I told J (midwife), she showed me the heartbeat on this side, so I was looking around here, and I couldn't find it, and I was thinking, "Oh here we go, I'm not going to be able to do this" . . . and my sister said, "Try the other side", and it was there straightaway . . . but now baby has settled down and it seems to be there at this side every time. As soon as I go on it I find it virtually straightaway . . .'

Continuity of care was considered very important:

'I like to know that it's the same midwife every time. That you can phone her up, send your trace, ask her things. I've asked her to do my delivery and she's agreed.'
'I don't want bossy midwives . . . but J is great, she lets you do it yourself.'

A longitudinal study of users' perspectives is occurring as part of the Valleys project. It is both quantitative and qualitative. Entitled What Pregnant Women Think, it aims to give users' views on service provision from the early antenatal period up to four months following delivery. Issues explored include:

- quality of care
- continuity of care
- patient held records
- parentcraft education
- degree of employer support.

A Valleys midwife described how users were taking the initiative in education provision:

'We have a family "drop in" centre in Abergavenny. We open enrolment for parentcraft sessions (we don't call them parentcraft, we call them antenatal support groups). The group decides their programme, virtually group discussion, a sort of group therapy. I think the midwives have actually developed themselves through this process; it's been a learning process for them, not just for the women. I've personally found it one of the most exciting things I've ever done.'

Researcher: 'What do members ask for?'

Midwife: 'They set the programme, but we look at how they feel about things, how they feel about coming to an antenatal clinic for the first time, and one girl who didn't contribute very much in the beginning, a very, very quiet little girl, came out with a statement: "I'm important . . ." and that's stuck with me for the last two years and I've thought that the girl has expressed the major problem we've got; we're trying to build up people's self-esteem and confidence.'

The future

All interviewees were asked about their hopes for the future. All users felt strongly that the service should continue and be expanded. Service providers were more concerned with service organization and resources.

One midwife referred to the review of midwifery services that had recently taken place in the UK:

'The Winterton Report recommends that we move to a community based maternity service . . . there should be midwifery units. DFM causes resource problems . . . we don't have enough community midwives to actually undertake DFM . . . it's very time consuming. So if we reorganize how we give maternity care in this area, if we integrate our midwifery service so that the majority of midwifery resources are actually based in the community, then I think DFM will be more effective because the resources will be there.' (Valleys Service Manager)

She then commented on cost effectiveness, saying:

'It's much better for patients because you're giving them the care in the home and it's better for us because we're not filling the hospital up with clinics with women waiting for long times (and) . . . we're not filling up hospital beds, so:

1 it gives a better quality of care to the woman

2 it's more cost effective, but we need more resources to do it . . . I hope the changes (to community provision) allow us to get them.'

Costs were also a major issue for the Valleys obstetrician:

'When we began, there were only three DFM systems going and it took a long time to evaluate and work out which was the best for us: none were perfect, even the one we use is not perfect, but it's better than the other two. Thereafter the most difficult thing was raising the money. We started with charitable monies . . . there is just not the capital in the NHS for such a scheme. We are constantly looking around and moving monitors from one place to another. We were fortunate to get six machines because we linked up with the Cardiff project and got some finance for our service needs . . . we've done it on a shoestring, which is why we have problems . . . we could probably do with twice as many machines . . . also, we haven't got the personnel to do it properly because our girls (midwives!) were already stretched before we introduced this, and by putting an extra burden on the community without increasing numbers, we are in danger of reducing quality.'

Quality was also an issue for a research midwife, who recognized the need for further training to develop her skills. The difficulties involved were voiced:

'The DFM course was just a basic study day . . . I want to go on more courses but getting finance to go on them . . . is very difficult. A day course is £30 then you would have to add travel and subsistence and cover for me while I'm away. I'd like a day going into the different types of traces and problems . . . purely on the technical side . . . different traces and different types of pregnancy . . . what's acceptable at 26–28 weeks, the relationship of trace to stage of gestation . . . also the effects of drugs on the fetus.

I've also been battling to go on a counselling course . . . a lot of women who have lost babies are very, very anxious . . . they've not really got over the previous loss before becoming pregnant again. You also need to relate to family problems . . . I'm often told by men that they feel left out . . . there are a lot of women and men out there who just feel that they're "going over the top", that's a common phrase they use, they're just coping . . . there's no need for it. We should be able to help them.'

The quality of both PHC services and the degree of teamwork was commented on by a Visiting Fogarty Fellow from the USA, who was in Wales to carry out a comparative study of the British and American systems for delivering obstetric and neonatal care:

'The common intellectual domain is almost identical between the two countries; I see very little difference, but they have taken quite radically different approaches in the way that they make sure that these become available to patients, ranging from the manpower and personnel that are used, to the organization and the inter-relationship between the units where women go. The most profound difference is the use of midwives. It is a profound difference and I'm quite persuaded that the system here is an excellent one . . . particularly when there are good inter-relationships with the practitioners representing the primary care sector and with the obstetrician representing the hospital sector . . . the primary care side of it here is absolutely outstanding.'

However, some interviewees saw problems for teamwork in the future. The attitudes of some service providers were particularly criticized:

> 'Different obstetricians have different views on the need. Some prefer to keep people in hospital . . . it's either all hospital or all community, not a sensible combination of both' (midwife)
>
> 'If hospital care is moved out into the community, the main battle will be with the obstetricians' (research team member)

Open access to care in the UK impressed the Visiting Fellow, as did the emphasis on prevention:

> 'In the States the major issue that we have struggled with, and written reams of papers about, is access to prenatal care and adequacy of prenatal care; here nobody understands the question because everybody has access. On the high tech side, no-one does it better than the States . . . America is the place of the numerators and the individual, not denominators, there is not really much attention to the population. You know, when that woman comes in who didn't get (primary health) care, we'll try to salvage her and her baby, but we don't have a system that prevents the thing from happening.'

However, consultant autonomy and the introduction of market principles in health care in the UK (and in Europe) dismayed him:

> 'I didn't expect each Unit to be doing its own thing. You do wonder, if you have a system like this (DFM) where potentially you could have some centralization, if there shouldn't be some recommendations from central Government, saying: these are the ones that we approve, recommend, and authorize, and we've worked out a special deal with the manufacturers to get you a price break.'

The Visiting Fellow was also very aware of the dangers of aggressive, competitive medical equipment marketing, and he sees this as a particular problem for European purchasers:

> 'Then there's the "gee whizz" factor . . . we've got this incredible thing . . . gee whiz, let's have one on the health service.'

Summary of domiciliary fetal monitoring

Quality

Domiciliary fetal monitoring, as part of an integrated domiciliary antenatal care scheme, is a model of good practice that can and should be extended to other antenatal care service organizations. It is effective, reflects a high degree of user responsiveness, is relatively cheap and easy to use, and is well accepted in practice by service providers and users.

The model of health on which care is based is social rather than exclusively medical, and the reorientation to PHC called for in the Ottawa Charter is evident. All service providers demonstrated a very clear and unanimous acceptance of a social model of health, and the way this applied to the particular circumstances of the patients they were seeing.

Continuity of care was an aspect that was very highly valued by patients. In the development of future schemes, this must be ensured.

Skills

With regard to skills, some staff believed that they would benefit from further training. One research midwife in particular spoke of the need to update both her technical and counselling skills. Meeting this need would be low cost in the short term (£30 for a one-day technical skills course) and could arguably save greater costs in the long term (eg from over-cautious hospitalizations or treatment of clinical depression in bereaved parents).

Costs

An evaluation of both the economic and social costs of the scheme is currently occurring, but the data obtained from this case study imply that DFM could be a more cost-efficient form of antenatal care for high risk pregnant women than hospitalization, with its attendant in-patient costs.

In addition to costs incurred by the health service, it is also necessary to take into account costs borne by families. There is no doubt that DFM is a lower cost solution for them than in-patient care. Whilst hard evidence about costs in both urban and rural areas is not yet available, all participants referred to the particular value of DFM in remote rural areas, where public transport is either poor or non-existent. Lack of transport has a 'knock on' effect for families when women are required to attend frequent out-patient appointments or be hospitalized (eg childcare, subsistence and visiting costs).

Teamworking

There was evidence of teamworking in both the Cardiff and the Valleys settings, but the ideal model (midwives, obstetricians and primary care teams collaborating) was the one known as the Cardiff Integrated Antenatal Care Scheme. In this, a common care management protocol had been agreed by the multidisciplinary team (hospital and community) and designated trained midwives were managing the scheme. The opportunity for implementation in the Valleys lies with the pending reorganization of midwifery services, which currently are separately based in the hospital and the community.

For teamwork to be effective, however, there needs to be a shared vision of care and the development and use of a care management protocol which recognizes and utilizes resources effectively. Indications are that some obstetricians and midwives will need to work more closely together to maximize the potential offered by DFM. This will necessitate attitude shifts in relation to:

- a more selective use of DFM.
- development of integrated care teams.
- two or more designated trained midwives to manage each DFM scheme.

Equity

Access to the scheme is equitable in that all those who are identified as having a high risk pregnancy, and who are able to benefit from DFM are offered it. Inequities nevertheless occur due to lack of equipment, especially telephones, in homes. This situation is recognized by service staff who go to great lengths to make the system work, often in the face of appalling odds.

For the purposes of preventive surveillance, a telephone is a medical appliance and should be treated as such. Telephones should be purchased and made available for loan for the duration of need, in the same way that any other piece of medical equipment is 'loaned' (wheelchair, walking frame, etc). As both high risk pregnancies and non-telephone ownership affect only a very small number of the total population of pregnant women, the cost will be low, and certainly cheaper than the cost of hospitalization.

Mobile telephones would be ideal for the purpose as neither installation nor disconnection costs would be accrued. It is worth noting here that Valleys midwives currently carry medical 'Pagers'. Provision of mobile telephones would allow them to send traces from homes when a telephone was not available. It would also be more efficient with regard to general service provision as they could be contacted immediately, thus time would not be lost finding a 'phone after being 'bleeped'.

Social integration

This issue is not relevant to this case study, as patients are monitored in their existing social setting with all their attendant support networks. For the patients' new role in life, however, (as mothers), midwives encourage the creation of new supportive social networks in the form of antenatal and parentcraft groups.

4 Telehealth and Adolescents

'. . . How do you like you so far?'

(service provider)

Type of service

Health promotion for adolescents.

Technology

An electronic Bulletin Board System (BBS). E ZOOT began as a one-line computer bulletin board system using a personal computer (PC) connected to a modem handling 2400 bps. The PC was donated by the telephone company. The operating software system was obtained free from a source in Toronto. It is called 'Shareware' and is easy to use.

Location

Edmonton (Canada).

Population

Adolescents.

Context

The decision to study health promotion with adolescents was prompted by the health potential they represent. They present our greatest opportunity for achieving a healthier future. These young people are the parents, citizens and leaders of tomorrow. Investing in them means investing in the future.

In choosing to look at an initiative operating in Canada the author recognized 'the moral and intellectual leadership that Canada has provided in the field of health promotion' (Cunningham, 1992).

The electronic BBS is called E ZOOT. It is one prong of a co-ordinated community education inter-agency approach by the Alberta Alcohol and Drug Abuse Commission (AADAC) (Jackson, 1992) to develop 'freedom, skills' in adolescents. It is complemented by initiatives such as *Two-way street: parents, kids and drugs*. This is a publication issued in co-operation with the Royal Canadian Mounted Police (RCMP), based on the recognition that most young people do not use drugs, but they are being called on to make their first decisions about them at an increasingly early age. One teenager wrote, in an Alberta essay contest:

> 'Teenagers want to be told that they are somebody and can be somebody without using drugs or alcohol. We want to be reassured of our place in life and know that we are accepted and deserve our parents' love.'

The objective of the personal development style of primary prevention is to empower people to do their own prevention. In this model, agencies do not do prevention to people – prevention doesn't happen until individuals do it. To be most effective, primary prevention needs to be global, rather than disease specific. This is recognized in the statement of E ZOOT design objectives (1987):

> 'prevention of intoxicant problems is not, and should not become, a major focus or priority . . . it is only one of the many hazards to be alert for.'

The level set for prevention work can also be problematic. If fixed too high, the preventee in a low risk situation will wonder what all the fuss is about, so fail to identify with the programme. If it is set too low, giving central life issues more weight, observers will wonder why a publicly funded addictions agency is doing all this 'human stuff'. This latter perspective will be a central concern of funding bodies, particularly during a time of both generalized economic recession and public spending cuts.

The position adopted by *AADAC* was to develop a framework that allows people to:

'move from the big picture to a specific focus, as the situation demands . . . (this way) individuals will be in a much better position to conduct their own prevention, priorities will be according to circumstance, and everyone will have a better idea of what the addictions agency is up to.' (E ZOOT Co-ordinator)

Technical description

E ZOOT is a multiline electronic Bulletin Board System (BBS) aimed at teenagers and young adults. It allows users to:

- leave public and private messages in over twenty areas
- review or download files containing information about alcohol, drugs and healthy lifestyles.
- upload or download public domain computer software.

The (24 hour) service is offered free within the Edmonton toll area. Most people in Alberta have access to a telephone and, apart from the low rental rate, local calls are free. E ZOOT is a member of five BBS message networks: SpiderNet, IMEXNet, DriftNet, FidoNet and WorldNet. User demand has been high, so in 1992 E ZOOT was upgraded to four incoming telephone lines/modems.

Health promotion information is collected by the systems operator and transcribed, then is available free to read or download. Health related queries raised by users are either answered by moderators direct or are networked to specific helping agencies, with information routed back through E ZOOT.

Moderators

Moderator volunteers from AADAC staff oversee discussions and keep them on track. All new users are subject to call-back verification to prevent obscenities being entered on the bulletin board (This was instituted after a problem in the summer of 1992.) A moderator describes the system:

'If we see an issue on the BBS of potential exploitation or a lurking adult with a negative motive . . . on one occasion we were very uncomfortable with what was going on and we called the police in, another occasion we had a young person who appeared to us to be suicidal, we worked that through and made sure that that young person got to the service required in order to remain safe.'

Service description

E ZOOT is offered by Community Education Services (CES), Edmonton, a prevention education unit of the AADAC. The goal is to serve programs aimed at increasing understanding, building personal competence, enhancing public awareness, and encouraging community action in the prevention of substance abuse.

A member of the team describes its origins:

'In 1981, AADAC undertook a very large multifaceted adolescent prevention campaign. It included an extensive media campaign that was funded in millions of dollars, on various different phases, over a 10 year period. As part of that, we also, undertook a refocus of what had been community extension services, into community education services, and that took on a very high primary prevention focus, particularly focused at the 12 to 17-year-olds, which we considered to be the youth population in Canada.

This project was quite unique in Canada. It emerged out of AADAC, embracing many of the principles of health promotion that were evolving at the time. This had many facets, including the evolution of peer support as an initiative and the development of a youth magazine called *Zoot Capri* that youths would receive in their homes; it was an adjunct to the school curriculum rather than distributed in school. Also, the AADAC had been sitting on curriculum development committees with Alberta Education for all levels: elementary, junior high and high school. There were particular aspects of alcohol and drug prevention initiatives in the curriculum, so there was development of curricula materials: posters, handout materials, a parent education component and an allied professional education component, so that teachers, nurses, counsellors and those involved with young people, would be included as well.

The context of *Zoot Capri* was to provide a health promotion vehicle that would, in a very subtle way, influence the behaviour of youths towards positive self-esteem, the development of skills and competences, and choice of health alternatives for behaviour that would increase the strength of the young person to withstand the pressures that would lead to dependence on alcohol and other drugs. So then, that came from a very positive perspective of empowering youth and the networks supporting youth.'

The youth population has changed:

'We did not have, until the last 10 years, an ethno-cultural mix in this part of the world . . . it was essentially white Anglo-Saxon Protestant, with some eastern European people and some small enclaves of Franco-Canadians and of course our aboriginal population, but we really didn't have much of a mix, and that's one of the reasons that the organization is beginning to look at ethno-cultural kinds of applications.' (team member)

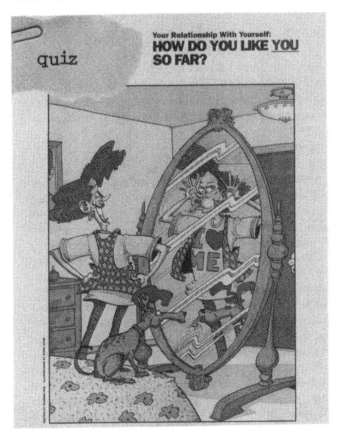

Figure 4: A cartoon from *Zoot Capri*

E ZOOT was started when the developers of the magazine *Zoot Capri* (an AADAC publication) began to look for a vehicle that was more interactive than the magazine. At the outset, there was an opportunity for innovation and visionary leadership:

> 'They put it out as an entrepreneurial gambit to the field and said, if you'll take over E ZOOT and let it run from 4.30 at night until 8.00 in the morning (the off hours), then you can have this computer equipment for in-house use in the daytime, to support your administrative function. We needed a computer, J had an interest in computers, we have always had a very strong youth prevention program team in this unit and we said we don't know a whole lot about this . . . but we finally decided, after much thinking, to set up an E ZOOT advisory committee of community partners to help us guide the process, and we adopted E ZOOT.' (team member)

The service is a reflection of the skills in the multidisciplinary team, which includes a psychologist, a church minister, an engineer, a social worker, a drama teacher, a cultural anthropologist and a food and nutrition specialist:

'We all seem to work together very well . . . there *is* no trained discipline to become an addictions counsellor; you can't do professional training to become an addictions counsellor . . . so the organization pulls from an eclectic group . . . that really embellishes the organization because people come from so many different agendas but focus on a similar set of principles and values.' (service manager)

It was recognized at the outset that the system would be used if it was adequately advertised and 'user friendly'. User friendliness poses a particular problem with regard to systems design. Generally, in computer generated activities, form rules function. When form rules, function can be both obscure and inaccessible, and thus demotivating for users. Process was a particularly relevant topic for E ZOOT designers as the goal of E ZOOT is to enhance the 'freedom skills' of users. This means handing over control in both the process (encouraging 'browsing'), and content (encouraging personal autonomy).

Specific objectives of E ZOOT are to:

- communicate the AADAC message via a youth-relevant Bulletin Board System (BBS)

- encourage users to develop communication and reasoning skills in an environment which allows for freedom of personal expression

- provide confidential, on-line counselling and/or referrals to appropriate agencies as requested or desired

- give CES and AADAC staff greater accessibility to the issues most relevant to youth today

- profile AADAC, E ZOOT and BBS technology to other helping communities

- monitor and document the effectiveness of BBS technology as a prevention initiative.

In North America, access to a telephone is less problematic than in Europe, and with the exception of public payphones, local calls are free. Access to PCs, however, may be more difficult. Recognizing this, AADAC staff and the Telephone Pioneers of North America assisted in setting up three donated PCs in youth clubs in two deprived city areas, and in the Adolescent Treatment Centre in Edmonton.

There is evidence of thorough and collaborative evaluation:

'Mental Health Services did a survey a couple of years back and asked kids where they would go for help for suicide, unplanned pregnancy, mental health or family problems, and they put AADAC for practically everything.'

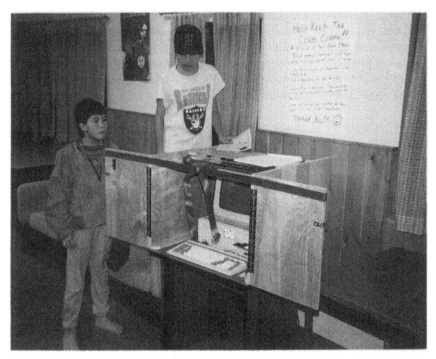

Figure 5: Children receiving a donated computer

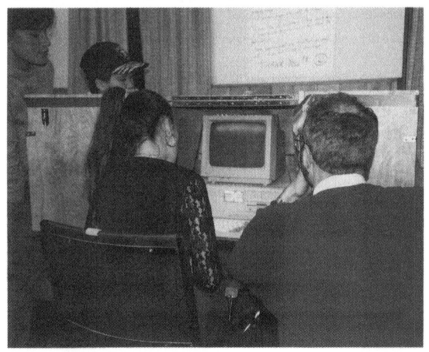

Figure 6: Youth using a new computer

The format is also seen as accessible:

> 'It was a real motivator for kids . . . they're already interested in computer technology, they're the ones who play Nintendo, get into computer games, and for them it's a motivating way to reach them . . . I mean, kids in grade 2 class in South Edmonton are talking to friends all over the world via computer. Unlike ourselves, who have had to become acquainted with it in our middle years (which is easier for some than it is for others!), these kids are growing up seeing this as a naturally available tool and if we just continue to provide posters and print material and so forth, we are eventually going to get behind the times.' (service manager)

Users

Due to E ZOOT's promise of anonymity, very little demographic information relating to users is held. However, it is known that most users are between the ages of 14 and 18-years-old, and most (85%) are male. It is interesting to note, however, that this is a smaller than the average sex split for use of bulletin boards. E ZOOT's annual report (Jackson, 1992) notes that figures for other BBSs are all over 90% male.

Users generate message threads. A message thread is defined as reciprocal message exchanges of three or more messages between two or more BBS users in which a common theme or topic is developed and discussed. A message thread begins when a new topic for discussion is introduced. It is fully underway once there are two or more related replies to the initial message. It has concluded once there can no longer be found any messages which relate to the initial topic. A message thread can also be considered complete if its topic has evolved to a point where it is no longer related to the initial topic. When this occurs, a starting point for a new thread should easily be identifiable.

Three hundred and two messages from the message area 'relationships' were collected over a five-week period (February 5th to March 10th 1992). 22 separate message threads were identified from the 302 messages. These included conversations related to gender, sexuality, help with meeting girls/women, the perfect relationship, rape and alcohol. Of the 22 identifiable message threads, 17 began as a request by a user for advice or information, while seven began through the introduction of a new topic by a participant. Continuation of the message thread depends on the reaction of the advice seeker to the comments of the advice giver(s).

Message threads take on three structural forms:

- linear – reciprocal message exchanges between two users

- linear parallel – advice seeking exchanges between users and the moderator

- complex – one or more discussions between multiple users.

Continued participation of the topic initiator is not necessary for the continued discussion of the issue. A complex message thread shows a greater willingness to engage in open conflict. Complex threads are shaped by topics which allow for, and encourage, open uninhibited debate.

One message thread began rather innocuously in the 'relationships' area when a user named Mary asked, 'How does alcohol affect someone's life?'. This simple question generated a heated debate totalling 37 responses and reactions over a 13-day period. Including the moderator, 12 users took part in the discussion.

Three replies were sent to Mary, and her six word question was her single contribution to the entire message thread.

Users are extremely inventive in their use of noting and using what are normally regarded as 'non-verbal' elements of communication in their verbal messages (see the smile:-) in Figure 7. A typical message might be: 'I didn't mean to SHOUT (grin)'. It is a common practice for BBS users to create

---

By Aquaman
To Deadhead
Re Alcohol

'Are you saying that if (your friend) drank his life would be full of excitement and fervour? Like hell. You are so often mentioning "dependency" in terms of relationships and how it is so crippling, yet you present yourself as being dependent on alcohol for all your social needs.'

By Deadhead
To Aquaman
Re Alcohol

'Hee hee, alcohol is a positive part of my life, just like 90% or so of the rest of the population. I present myself as dependent? I'd like some proof of that. Since you will have a real hard time finding proof, let me give you some: . . . OH I NEED BOOZE, I NEED BOOZE BAD, I CAN'T LIVE WITHOUT IT . . . There you go . . . :-) (note smile) . . . For ALL my social needs? Whadya mean? So socially, all I need is a bottle? Please prove it noble sir. My social life is unbounded, unlike some people I know . . .'

Figure 7: Part of a message thread about alcohol

'smilies' through combinations of keyboard characters, to punctuate/illustrate points that they are trying to make. These need to be viewed by turning this page sideways – *see* Figure 8.

:-)	=	smiling face
;-)	=	wink and smiling face
:-(	=	sad face
d:-)	=	Smiling face with baseball cap
B-)	=	smiling face with glasses

Figure 8:   'Smilies'

Bulletin Boards are rich in social interaction:

'Until recently, the notion that social and or cultural data could exist in the computer mediated communications (CMC) context has been overlooked or discounted.' (Jackson, 1993)

Jackson goes on to quote a study by Myers (1987) in which it was found that the CMC environment of an electronic BBS could be seething with an abundance of social activity. Myers' findings reveal that a unique form of interaction exists and the BBS messages provide an ideal forum for uninhibited, anonymous communication which is particularly valuable for teenagers.

The team were asked whether they thought use of a BBS limited social interaction:

'Kids at dances are a lot more involved with one another because of knowing one another via the BB, many set up meetings to get together, once they get to know each other on the BB they want to meet each other and get together. For those who don't want that they can still reach out, this is a faceless person you are meeting on the BB, but not a cold medium, actually a very warm medium in the sense that people needing to can reach out.' (team member)

'The way it's offered is another form of empowerment . . . boys' and girls' clubs having problems keeping teen (age) members, wherever an E ZOOT has been located they are pulling those teens back and the kids can't always get onto the BB straightaway . . . so other dialogue is going on while they are waiting to get on to the (one) computer in the club . . . discussions are going on re staying in school, family problems . . . so the BB is like a carrot that tempts the teens back into the clubs.' (service manager)

The future

The researcher talked with E ZOOT organizers about the future. There is now a solid core of regular system users and many calls for extension of the service have been made. For these to be met, more resources are needed, plus a new computer with a greater capacity and handling speed:

'Our success has been one of our blocks in the way; it's grown so fast, and it's got so much potential that it could consume this entire unit.' (service manager)

J agrees: 'We're in a time in Alberta when our Government is trying to manage a debt, and as a Government Agency, we feel accountable to that situation; also as tax paying citizens we do, but here you have a really incredible potential and to keep it reigned in has been quite a challenge.'

Another desired change is that the needs of community partners, as opposed to individual users, should be made a priority. It is recommended that two additional dedicated telephone lines be added in youth clubs in two other downtown areas.

The heavy use of E ZOOT by males and its underuse by females is a source of concern, but the team have seen the user gap narrow (slowly) over the last two years. It is believed that provision of computers in youth centres, with support for female use encouraged by staff, will help the shift. Teachers are also aware of the problem and are working on it with AADAC. The *Zoot Capri* magazine also promotes the use of the Bulletin Board and positive messages to build the self-esteem of young females.

Summary of E ZOOT

Quality

E ZOOT is an outstanding example of good practice. Service quality and relevance are demonstrated by increase in use and demand, and by both 'in-house' and external service evaluation. A social model of health is used and exploited to its full potential. All of the HFA principles enshrined in the Ottawa Charter are evident. Service provision has been reoriented towards community responsive health promotion, and the creation of supportive environments for the making of healthy lifestyle choices is evident, as is collaboration with other providers and networks to develop healthy public policy.

Skills

The skills of both providers and users have grown. Service providers possess a wide range of skills and these are pooled and extended by teamwork. This allows a coherent shared vision of service provision to develop. The openness and flexibility of the E ZOOT team spills over into the way users experience the system. There is evidence of development of ongoing self-esteem amongst users, reflected in the way decisions about health risks such as alcohol use are handled.

Costs

Costs are very low. Donated and reconditioned PCs have been used, donated software was traded, and the network expanded. Four Modems cost less than 800 CD (480 ECU). Staff costs have increased only slightly (a systems operator has been employed), but existing staff have shifted priorities to run E ZOOT.

The service began modestly; planned growth is also modest, in line with the quality of service staff know they can deliver within budget limitations. It is gratifying to note that, although AADAC has suffered a budget cut, E ZOOT work has been protected.

The team have achieved much with limited resources. Their success must be seen as largely due to the existence of an open management style, in which risks are taken, creativity is supported and everyone's contribution is valued.

Teamworking

A large part of E ZOOT's success is due to teamworking. Not only do the team model good intra-team skills, they also model good extra-team skills in the way they work with other organizations (eg schools, parents, police) to build a shared vision of the health potential of young Albertans.

Equity

Service access is not a major problem for the population served. Many young people have home computers, and in areas of deprivation computers have been made available in schools and youth centres. The fact that local telephone calls are free must help enormously.

Ethical issues were quite problematic to the team, who gave a lot of thought to how they could moderate use, yet have the BBS belong to the users. The system they have evolved, of roving moderators, together with a call-back verification facility, seems to be working well.

Social integration

Contrary to the widely held belief that use of technology promotes social isolation, E ZOOT was found to promote social interaction. This was true not only of interaction using the technology alone, but use of the technology also sometimes prompted people to agree to meet each other socially.

5 Telehealth and Disability

'a ship to carry a mouse'

(service provider)

Type of service

Information system for disabled people.

Technology

CD-ROM based information system (HANDYNET). HANDYNET is a DG V (HELIOS) project to establish a Europe wide information system on all aspects of living with a disability. HANDYNET information is provided on a database using a CD-ROM format. A new compact disc is produced three times a year. Other communications are via an electronic newsletter and an electronic mail facility to active partners in the system.

Location

All EU countries participate. The Netherlands and Italy were visited.

Population

Disabled people.

Context

The objective of HANDYNET is to promote independence for disabled people through improved access to information about topics such as daily living equipment, leisure, travel and employment. The target audience is professionals and disabled people themselves.

Funding services for disabled people is an issue which concerns all EU countries. A national debate, 'Choices in Health Care,' began in 1992 in The Netherlands (*see* the report published by the Ministry of Health on Choices in Health Care in 1992). Its intention is to promote public discussion of issues concerning choice and public responsibility in health care. The report addresses issues relevant to all EU countries, indeed all Western countries, and is principally concerned with 'value for money' in health care:

> 'One important reason why choices are necessary is that the population is ageing, which leads to a growing demand for health care and a need for more care for the chronically ill . . . Another reason is that scientific and technological change is rapid and attracts funding and publicity. At the same time, financial choices are limited.'

In addition to the elderly (who may become disabled through chronic disease), the disabled population in Europe is estimated to be 10% in the EU member states. Social trends in Europe indicate the likelihood of decreased collective taxation, so choices will have to be made about what services and products are needed, and are socially and economically 'worth' providing. This raises issues such as the prioritization and the rationing of services and products, and the need to control and evaluate innovations more carefully. HANDYNET, as a Europe wide technology project for disabled people, was therefore selected for study.

The main area of activity is in developing the database. It is organized into the following modules:

- Technical Aids
- Vocational Training
- Employment
- Accessibility
- Leisure.

Work is progressing on the first pilot module (Technical Aids). Council decision 93/136/EEC decrees that work on other modules should not begin until the Technical Aids module is complete.

Each Member State has nominated a co-ordination agency to collect and disseminate information in their country. Data collection has been assisted by the acceptance and use of the ISO (International Standards Organization) classification system on equipment for disabled people. The material currently stored is mainly an extensive catalogue of technical aids (medical equipment).

HANDYNET was originally conceived as a traditional on-line database with phone-up access through modems and terminals or personal computers. The change to CD-ROM is said to open up new possibilities as more information can be stored. In addition to possessing the necessary hardware, information systems need to be 'user friendly'. They should be easy to use with minimal instruction, and the content should not require prior subject knowledge. HANDYNET planners have sought to meet these requirements by choosing a simple operating program for manipulating data (Windows, operated by a mouse or a communication aid). In addition, all nine EU languages are available. Users are asked which language they wish to use, and all subsequent prompts appear in that language.

Case study visits were made to The Netherlands and Italy.

HANDYNET: The Netherlands

The Netherlands has been operating a policy of integration rather than segregation with regard to disability in society. Currently equipment is provided free of charge to users. It is funded by National Basic Health Insurance. Provision can be made through a number of routes. Employers, employees, government and organizations (such as The Netherlands Independent Living Movement) are involved in decision making.

The Netherlands, like other European countries, is introducing market principles into provision of health care. This has implications for the provision of technical aids and services. Health assurance companies or funds will be the purchasers. They will negotiate with producers and service providers. According to Bougie (1991), technical aids will be a small part of the whole package, and 'open ended' budgets will cease to exist.

Service description

The data collection centre in The Netherlands is the Revalidatie Informatie Centrum (RIC) at Hoensbroek. RIC is part of Lucas Stitching voor Revalidatie. The centre has expertise in the use of CD-ROM to store and handle data.

RIC was founded in 1961 as a nursing home and rehabilitation centre. It is now a large rehabilitation clinic, housing a number of associated centres. It is responsible for providing information on a wide range of information topics and on the welfare of physically handicapped people. The centre is used mainly by rehabilitation professionals, community workers and disabled people. There is an extensive resource centre, including on-line search facilities, extensive product documentation facilities, and an exhibition room where a large number of technical aids are available for viewing and trial. The centre co-operates with others at a number of levels: provincial, national and international.

Associated Hoensbroek centres offer the following services/facilities:

- rehabilitation
- audiology
- vocational training

- a large sports complex
- a gardening area for disabled people
- the Institute for Rehabilitation Research (IRV).

The HANDYNET co-ordinator describes The Netherlands history of collaborating with HANDYNET:

'We started out in the beginning for the information provision of our country. Now we have our own large database (HANDYNET is part of it) . . . there were big differences in the beginning in Europe, and HANDYNET is based on the shared way of work and so it is not only here but in all Member States; that's not easy to get all these things organized and arranged, it costs a lot of time. (But) the system exists now and it has a lot of very reasonable and interesting information on it. HANDYNET does not give the one and only and the best solution by definition, but it is a tool with which you have possible solutions (to choosing technical aids) and the users should be able to do a good assessment.'

He went on to discuss other modules that could address activities of daily living with disability, and the following example from RICs own database was quoted:

'We add a structure which gives the differences between products which have more or less the same function. For example, a spoon was produced in one country and distributed to another country and the spoon had a name, like the spoon for handicapped people. The same spoon came by another channel to that same country and it was called the spoon for left-handed people. The third time we found that same spoon was in our own country and it was called an adaptable spoon. This spoon had come with three different descriptions, three different target groups, three different prices and three different suppliers, but it was the same product. What we can add is that it is one and the same product.'

Users

With regard to information for users, the HANDYNET co-ordinator said:

'Of course we get reactions like . . . why doesn't the file, the system . . . contain more information on products, and not only the reference that the product exists, and the place where you can get it. We understood the comments and studied how we could enlarge the data . . . to enable the user to go one step further than only the reference to the commercial

brochure . . . further investigations showed that this would be a tre-
mendous problem of time and money to collect the data and to update the
data on the products. We communicated our views with other HANDYNET
centres in other countries . . . and the conclusion was that we are not alone
in this problem.'

The problem of lack of user involvement and user relevance associated with
HANDYNET is not an RIC one, but one that was designed into HANDYNET
at the outset. RIC is very user aware and user friendly and has resources which
could be included in HANDYNET, should it be invited to work on another
module than Technical Aids.

An example of the degree and type of social integration offered by RIC is
found in both the centre itself, and educated provision for young disabled
people. Disabled people can stay at the RIC centre, or visit on an out-patient
basis. The idea of providing assessment, rehabilitation, education and leisure
opportunities all in one setting is that users can have the opportunity to be
supported while they learn to become fully integrated members of society.

Of special interest is the Vocational Education Centre for young people.
Disabled students from all over the Netherlands come to study at the centre.
They follow a two-year course and are awarded a National Certificate upon
successful completion. A residence is provided, comprising individual flats.
90% of students are reported to find jobs following graduation.

The future

Regarding the future, the co-ordinator had views on how the Technical Aids
module might progress, and the need for further training for service providers:

'About the user information: it is obvious that information on the use and
user of the product is very important . . . it is not easy to collect those data,
but HANDYNET is very interested in going in that direction in future. What
we decided to do for the time being is to refer to existing literature in that
field, the product description gives a reference to literature and documentation on evaluation and we have references to official standards, which is
another type of evaluation; it's more laboratory tests . . . the other development is training. It starts with the basic education of the professionals of the
future . . . secondly we have to do a lot of work in postgraduate training,
where tools like information systems have to be introduced to a lot of people
. . . Several times a year we offer a course for professional therapists,
'Handicap and Technology' . . . the scope of the course is, how can
technology be used by handicapped people? and HANDYNET is one of the
things we introduce in that course, in the context of one tool in the
assessment procedures.'

The Netherlands Independent Living Movement

The Independent Living Movement originated in the 1980s, in Berkley, California. What started as a group of students 'standing up for their rights', turned into a political movement. The philosophy spread to Europe and the European Network for Independent Living (ENIL) was formed. Independent Living was set up in The Netherlands in 1989. Its goal is the emancipation of people with disabilities. The main areas of activity include:

- peer counselling to build the self-respect of disabled people

- support for people who take legal actions relating to disability issues

- lobbying for client-linked budgets so that disabled people can make their own living, work and leisure choices

- publicity related activities to raise the profile of disabled people and to ensure their emancipation.

Two members of the Independent Living Movement were interviewed in the home of one of them (a wheelchair user). They were asked about their involvement with HANDYNET:

'For me . . . it's a very strange thing, it is remote. I hear about it from EC conferences and hear nice speeches and you can read in the HELIOS magazine about it, but it doesn't live for us. The (NIL) office in Rotterdam has software from the national information centre, and our own software for the region, but they don't know HANDYNET at all. It's not really available for the consumers; my organization is a consumer organization.' (user 1)

She went on to describe the organization's data collection activities:

'My organization has done some research on need for information of disabled, elderly, and foreigners living here . . . and found that when you ask for information you have to start with the needs of the people, and say: what is the way that people ask for information, how can you fit it in your (information) network? . . . technical aids, it doesn't fit, it doesn't fit at all. I've also been secretary of an organization that for more than 10 years has tried to get more information on technical aids . . . this is an organization run by consumers themselves and research people. They said: . . . together we know a lot. How can we research other information to help people choose the best that is available at the moment? (but) we got nothing from the Government to do the research . . .'

Researcher: 'So where do you start from, the normal everyday things that we all do, like me finding your home?'

User 2: 'Yes, that's the right question to ask . . . I think they started HANDYNET before asking (us) those questions first . . . first they start with a computer, and the technical people who say, oh we can put lots of information in that, instead of thinking what sort of information do disabled people need.'

User 1: 'If I know someone in the country (being visited) I phone and say I need . . . for example, when we go to Prague we know someone there and we call and ask them what's the best place to stay, what are costs, what's the best way, to fly or by car, or by train and so on. Then you see the costs and you make your own choice and then you need information about accessibility, and if by plane, is it possible to take your wheelchair with you, and if the electric wheelchair gives you a lot of problems then you get an ordinary wheelchair, then you need a paper that says you can take the chair in the plane with you and not in the luggage, that kind of thing. . . . last week I was contacted in Rotterdam by a woman in a wheelchair who got my name from the help desk at Schipol (airport), there is a help desk there for disabled people . . . it's a good system, when you know it.'

The discussion moved on to the future. The main concern was with the outcome of the reorganization and refinancing of health and social care that is currently taking place in The Netherlands. It was believed that the rights of disabled people were under threat.

User 1: 'I think we have had a good system in The Netherlands for disabled people, we can get our houses adapted, grants for taxis or for own car, but with a new law which starts next year it seems to us that all provisions are breaking down . . . provision was available for those up to 65 years (old) . . . now the law is changing to include those over 65 . . . I think that's very good. But this means that the number of people qualifying for aid is double what it was. Also, with the move to decentralization, the Government is cutting a third of the money (so twice the number of disabled have only two thirds of the current allocation). Also, now you can only get support for a car if you have a job, so you become doubly disadvantaged. Since decentralization the local spending has been on public transportation . . . this often means five or six disabled people being transported in one bus and that's segregation, it's not what we want . . . it's going back in time; we didn't want it then!'

Researcher: 'How do you make your views known?'

User 1: 'We have the National Council of the Disabled, they are in discussion with the umbrella of the communities and the parliament, then the local organizations, like mine in Rotterdam. We are just working together with the national level, we are also working with the regional organizations (to promote pressure at the national level). We have 12 provinces and each one has a national agency for the policy of disabled people. We work strongly together. All we do in the locality, we report to the province and the province brings it together at the national level.'

Review

The presentation of data for The Netherlands has been deliberately wide ranging in order to illustrate the opportunities that exist for compilers of information systems. A summary of the HANDYNET system follows the next HANDYNET case study.

What is clearly evident from the data collected in The Netherlands is that a great deal of good practice (in the form of skills, expertise and experience) is available, and a large number of resources exist which HANDYNET is not making use of. Most striking is the lack of involvement of users in the system. Whilst a real need exists, which could be addressed, the two systems (HANDYNET and the Independent Living Movement) operate in isolation of each other. Not only is this a shameful waste of resources, it is ethically indefensible.

HANDYNET: Italy

Italy is a rapidly 'greying' country. Its population has the fourteenth highest proportion of the elderly worldwide. Owing to the current zero population growth, it will leap to the top of the list by the year 2000, with nearly 10 million people over 65-years-old. This demographic shift will influence the need for services for the disabled.

The Italian Government is politically unstable at the time of writing, but trends evident in other EU countries also apply to Italy, such as the introduction of market principles into health and welfare provision, and the move towards care in the community.

The perceptions of an Israeli psychologist, working at the HANDYNET co-ordinating centre in Milan, are interesting. She recalls that, when she first came to Italy, six years previously, she never saw disabled people in public places:

> 'It was as if they were all hidden away. Now you see them all over the place, for example there is a law that says that a certain number of the workforce of large companies must be from the disabled. Also there are no special schools . . . disabled children are integrated into normal schools.'

Three settings in northern Italy were visited: the national co-ordinating centre (SIVA) in Milan, an information centre in Cadore, and the PRISMA centre in Belluno.

Service description

SIVA (Servizio Informatzioni e Valuatazione Ausili) Technical Aids Information and Testing Centre is a section of the Bio-engineering Centre of the Pro Juvetute Foundation in Milan. SIVA is the national co-ordinating centre for HANDYNET. Activities include the development, management and distribution of a computerized information system, research programmes, a testing laboratory, and an information and advice service.

The advice service is run by a team which includes two occupational therapists, three physiotherapists with experience on technical aids, one computer technician and a secretary. The basic tools which support the work of the team are:

- SIVA's own computerized information system
- a specialized library with literature, paper files and audiovisuals
- a permanent exhibition of technical aids.

The service is open every weekday morning. Advice is provided mainly upon appointment, by mail or on the telephone. One member of the team is always available to answer telephone queries from clients who seek advice. Clients may be referred by a health or welfare worker, or may refer themselves. A consultation starts with a discussion with the client in order to focus his/her perceived problem with reference to the situation and expectations. In most cases, the consultation is carried out by a single member of the team who is on duty. In principle, each member of the team is able to respond to any request. At regular intervals a 'follow up' inquiry is performed on samples of clients who have received services six to 12 months previously. A standardized form is mailed, asking for information on possible actions undertaken after SIVA's recommendations. Data processing through the same software provides an insight into the effectiveness of the service in meeting the clients' need (Andricht and Pedotti, 1992).

The SIVA model has been disseminated throughout Italy in a number of ways;

- publication of guidelines for Technical Aids information centres in Italy
- design and development of a regularly updated educational programme for Technical Aids advice:
  - **Module 1** Basics of technical aids for independent living
  - **Module 2** Training on computerized information systems
  - **Module 3** Advising on technical aids.

Discussions took place with the HANDYNET co-ordinator about the early experiences of working on HANDYNET, and its future direction:

'(At the beginning) it was very difficult work, even when at first there were only three of us . . . there were three ways of thinking, three different professional backgrounds, technical . . . computermen. We had experience of running an information system so had a certain structure in mind . . . so there was the need to create a consensus of people from different countries or different backgrounds. The structure grew very complicated, and testing proved this, so the second stage was a process of refinement; a level of consensus was arrived at and work began to spread to other countries. The introduction of HELIOS (as an umbrella organization) made things very much simpler (contact was on tap in Brussels from then). Technology was growing faster than HANDYNET at that time, so things had to be reformatted for PCs (and) . . . every step had to be vetted by some consultative committee or other, even after HELIOS . . . we were slowed down by the political process. Another thing was the contract for software going to a space agency who knew nothing about our previous work . . . it was like using a ship to carry a mouse. When HELIOS started, there was management . . .'

On the issue of who HANDYNET was for, he clearly saw it as a resource for professionals:

'If I go to buy a car, I go to the showroom and ask the salesmen all the technical details (but) . . . of course when we speak of professionals as advisers we may also be talking about the disabled themselves.'

Whoever uses the system it was strongly advocated that a supportive educational infrastructure be kept in place. SIVA offers courses on all its services to disability health workers. Courses are open to all, throughout Italy. Attendance is credited and participants are kept on a mailing list for newsletters and further meetings. SIVA has been invited by the HANDYNET co-ordinator in Greece to advice on setting up a similar system there.

It was believed that the Technical Aids module could be strengthened in the future by adding users' views on products and services. A large, thick file exists on evaluation and information that has been sent in across the years by users. It was recognized, however, that it would take time and money to adapt this information into a form in which it could be readily accessed by users.

Now the HANDYNET technology and network existed it could develop more quickly and in a more exciting way. The service centre at Belluno (The Dolomites) was cited as a good resource for developing a future HANDYNET module on leisure for disabled people.

CADORE local information centre

The area of Cadore has 30 000 inhabitants; it has good transportation access to main towns, but includes a vast mountainous area (the Dolomites) where transport and communication problems can be severe. It is also an international tourist area and, as such, receives a lot of temporary visitors.

In the Cadore team, each person has 20 children in their care, dealing with all problems, including physiological, psychomotor and psychological (not just disabled). They give advice on technical aids to all citizens. About three times a year the team meet with schoolteachers to identify children with a suspected disability. Thereafter they attend multidisciplinary case conferences regularly (families also attend). After 16 years of age, vocational training is given to enable the disabled person to enter the job market. This is networked from schools, medical centres and employment agencies. The law requires of companies that 6% of their employees should be drawn from the registered disabled. There has been a recent local development of social co-operatives in which 60% of employees are able-bodied and 40% are disabled.

Staff were asked how they thought an information system could help. They had no experience of HANDYNET, so replies are based on use of SIVA SYST. Here are some replies:

'You get information. It offers a wider range of possibilities for overcoming disability and reducing resistance to disability. For example, the pilot scheme in Genoa and Bologna during the three-year mid-school period is a good model. Some work experience takes place and also specific training for disability. This type of thing is now significantly changing employer attitudes to disability, opening doors (and minds) to change.' (psychologist)

'We can get details of all the latest equipment, courses and information, otherwise we're in danger of being very isolated.' (physiotherapist)

'We use it more than the other staff, but it is only a part of what we do. We have the older (floppy) version of SIVA SYST, we can't afford a new PC or CD-ROM for the latest version.' (service manager)

The local co-ordinator here interjected with the information that only yesterday he had met with local administration officials to explore reasons for a recent budget cut. Reasons given were economic. The co-ordinator had made the point that use of an information system could save money in the long run (health promotion).

The researcher explored the value of having a European information system. Everyone was emphatic that they could see no negative consequences, but most thought that a module on technical aids was fairly limited in its applicability; modules should be extended to include information on holidays, work and leisure.

Users: Centro Studi PRISMA (Belluno)

From November 1988 to December 1991, PRISMA was acknowledged by the EC as one of 32 local model activities (LMA) for social integration of the disabled, (network III of the HELIOS programme, Social Integration and Co-ordination).

PRISMA, founded in 1984, is a cultural association of people (some disabled, some working in the field) from various parts of Italy, who are concerned with disability and social integration:

'The association aims at promoting culture and information concerning all the aspects of medical and social rehabilitation. The idea behind this is the

conviction that dissemination of scientific, wide ranging and interdisciplinary information is the necessary basis for fostering the removal of social,
cultural and technical barriers which hinder full participation of disabled
persons in society.' (PRISMA bylaws, item 2)

PRISMA uses an interdisciplinary approach. Physicians, therapists, social
workers and educators concerned with the disabled are involved. Architects,
engineers, teachers, tourism professionals, technicians, designers, civil ser-
vants, employers and many other professionals are also given the opportunity
to be directly involved in the integration process. Above all, the disabled
person's direct experience of disability is recognized as the main professional
resource.

The Manager of PRISMA is **G**. This is his story:

'I had an accident in Arabia six years ago. I was a clerk of works in a building
firm, the accident made me paraplegic.'

G's wife, who also works for PRISMA, adds: 'He had been collecting
information on technical aids before he came to PRISMA. I got him to go
on the first course. He was very, very reluctant.

Researcher asks: 'Why were you reluctant?'

G replies: 'Shame. Ashamed to go outside of home.'

The course was only a year after his accident but he met **R** (HANDYNET
co-ordinator), who involved him in drawing up plans (using his building
knowledge) for a holiday centre for the disabled. Figure 9 shows his design
for a sports area for disabled people. **G** continues to do building drawings
and now has a special drawing board at home purchased by a private
foundation fund, '. . . so after this I was almost obliged to do something.'

The PRISMA course and experience convinced him about social integration and the need to disseminate his experience to other disabled people. He
is now one of the teachers on the PRISMA courses and took part in the second
and third of the first level courses.

Researcher 'What makes you a special teacher?'

G: 'I was a professional before, also my personal condition makes me study
solutions, not only for me but for others like me.'

G's wife: 'The first thing he asked for after the accident was for a pen, to
do some work.'

In addition to maintaining a library and information service for the disabled
at local, regional and national level, PRISMA is the organizer of a number of
courses, congresses and other initiatives such as:

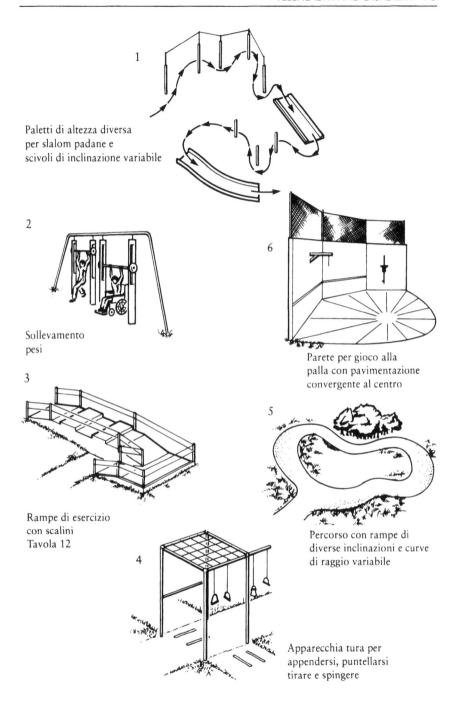

Figure 9: Design for a sports centre for disabled people. Reproduced from *Handicap E Vacanze. Accessibilita delle Strutture Turistiche, Centro Studi Prisma,* Fondazione Don Aldo Belli, Instituto Bellunese Di Ricerce Sociali E Culturali, p. 15. Serie 'Varie' n.15 (1987)

- a documentation centre
- an information advice service on independent living
- education for independent living – residential courses
- education of schoolchildren about disability
- transport and driving legislation
- accessibility to the natural environment.

PRISMA organized the first national congress on 'Handicap and holidays: accessibility and touristic facilities', and has now undertaken a study concerning the accessibility of the disabled person to the natural environment. A guide to mountain paths tested as accessible to wheelchair users has been published (*Dieci proposte di Itinerari accessibili nell'Alpago*) (*see* Figure 10).

Similar initiatives have been suggested to other regions and there has been an impressive response. Increasingly, PRISMA is being recognized as a centre for demonstration of good practice in promoting the health and well-being of disabled people. Two of their initiatives are described below.

Education for independent living – residential courses

In the mountain village of Cortina d'Ampezzo, PRISMA has offered courses on a summer residential basis, available to disabled persons from all over Italy. There are two modules, each a week long:

- Disability and Daily Life: education toward independent living
- Disability and Society: promoting independent living.

The programme of the first course deals with dependency as a way of approaching life and coping actively with disability, with the understanding that nobody in the world is fully independent, but that all of us are in some way dependent on each other.

The disabled person is trained to gain awareness of the value of their own experience and practise the ability to rationalize it and make use of it for counselling other disabled persons in achieving a better quality of life. This concept is further exploited in the second level course in which the participants learn and exchange techniques and methods for relating to other people with different disabilities, for managing information, and for using the mass media as a vehicle for promoting positive attitudes in society with regard to disability.

6

Strada delle Malghe

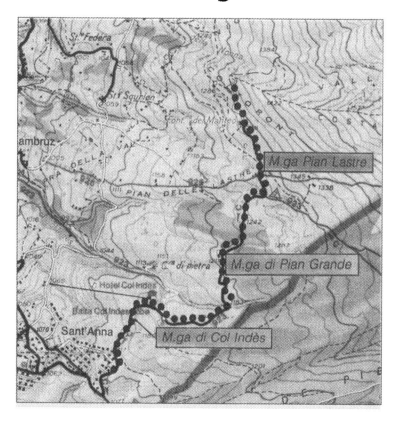

CARATTERISTICHE TECNICHE

Tempo di percorrenza: 2 ore (lunghezza circa m 2.500).
Difficoltà: nessuna. Percorso interamente asfaltato, percorribile da qualsiasi carrozzina con pendenza media inferiore all'8%.

22

Figure 10: Strada delle Malghe (de *Dieci proposte di itinerari accessibili nell'Alpago*)

Education of schoolchildren about disability

From 1989 to 1991, PRISMA developed an experimental project in primary schools concerning the 'education of schoolchildren to correct attitudes towards disabled persons'. This was approved by the Ministry of Education and was implemented in a large number of schools. The project aimed to develop in the able-bodied children the ability to establish relationships with persons with disability, consider the value of the person beyond disability, and understand the physical and psychological barriers which exist in society, and how they can be removed. The results and findings of the project have been published in a book which is being introduced into primary schools.

Review

In Italy, as in The Netherlands, good practice in meeting the needs of disabled people exists in spite of rather than because of HANDYNET. The relationship between the national co-ordinating centre (SIVA) and the service centre (PRISMA) was found to be excellent, with evidence of close collaboration in the delivery of a high quality, responsive, user friendly service.

Service provision at PRISMA was found to be particularly democratic and imaginative, and to strongly reflect Health For All principles. PRISMA work should be vigorously promoted so that it is recognized and disseminated as a model of good practice.

Summary of HANDYNET

Quality

HANDYNET got off to a bad start. At the beginning, there was an overall lack of clarity about its role and potential, lack of shared vision, and lack of leadership.

In both its organization and its choice of pilot module (Technical Aids) there was evidence of autocratic 'Top down' organization. Choice of subject also meant that the model of health used was limited to the traditional medical model, yet evidence from case study locations indicated full and imaginative use of a user and community responsive social model.

Skills

In both countries, it was believed that a computerized information system was only one of a number of resources that should be offered to assist disabled people in their day-to-day lives. It was recognized that the database should be used as part of an integrated care system and that staff needed training in both the use of the system and the social skills that are needed when working with people.

Costs

It has not been possible to get full details of costs, but the length (began in 1986) and scale of HANDYNET work indicate that fairly substantial costs will have been involved. A better decision, with regard to effectiveness as well as efficiency, might have been to fund more collaborative pilot work in fewer countries on two modules. In addition to Technical Aids, for example, another module could have explored pan European social data, such as employment or leisure opportunities and legislation. In both instances, users and users' organizations would be involved at the outset and ongoing built in evaluation would be required.

Teamworking

Whilst a degree of teamworking between countries is evident, there was little evidence of teamwork involving other interested parties or groups. Since its creation, HELIOS has improved international teamworking.

Equity

As it stands currently, HANDYNET seems to be a scheme constructed by providers for providers. This is particularly regrettable in view of the good practice in service provision that was found to exist in the national host institutions.

Social integration

The current format (on its own) and the choice of module have not encouraged social integration. In addition to developing further models relating to the social, as opposed to the medical, aspects of everyday life, other formats such as the E Mail facility should be explored so that users can themselves enter and 'own' data, for example on product evaluations and work and leisure opportunities.

6 Telehealth and the Elderly

'. . . doing nicely at home . . .'

(user)

Type of service

Support for independent living.

Technology

This consists of alarm systems. An alarm system is an electronic system which allows elderly or disabled people living on their own to call for help by means of a signal which is received elsewhere, resulting in assistance being given. The alarm set is worked by means of a mobile transmitter, bell pull or push button. The service centre or the carers (neighbours, relatives or friends) then organize assistance, either by calling in services or going to the person's assistance themselves.

The Technology Initiative for Disabled and Elderly People (TIDE) is a research and development initiative aimed at stimulating the creation of a single market in rehabilitation technology in Europe. (TIDE Workplan 1993–94). Alarm/alert systems are being developed in TIDE project 141, 'Future alarm and awareness services for the disabled and elderly' (FASDE). At the time of the study, FASDE demonstration projects were occurring in The Netherlands, England, Germany, Spain and Sweden.

Location

Provision was explored in two different settings. The first was part of the EC TIDE initiative in The Netherlands, and the second was a voluntary service in Canada.

Population

Principally elderly people.

Context

In the year 2010, one in four people in Europe will be aged over 60, and can expect to experience perceptual defects (TIDE Workplan 1993–94). Most people continue independent living even when impairments develop. This is possible when the social, cultural and physical home environment facilitates independence.

The TIDE project is exploring 'state of the art' alarm provision for the elderly and disabled. A number of devices are on trial, including pendants, small 'clip on' alarms, and wrist-watch alarms.

Alarm systems: The Netherlands

As in the rest of Europe, the percentage of elderly people in The Netherlands will increase. More people than ever before will continue to live in their own homes. Government policy is aimed at a reduction of the percentage of elderly living in medical and non-medical institutional settings (currently about 11%). Emergency response systems (alarms) are considered as one of the ways to support independent living. About 3% of The Netherlands population have alarm systems.

Alarm devices are part of a group of provisions comprising home care technology aimed at the promotion of independent living. In The Netherlands, home care has been defined as:

> 'the entire system of care, nursing, treatment and counselling of clients living at home, that performs its task using self care, care by persons in the direct social environment, volunteer aid, and/or additional professional care'. (National Council for Public Health, The Netherlands, 1990)

In 1990, integration of alarm systems with medical and social services in The Netherlands was reported as far from complete (Institute for Rehabilitation Research internal document). This is partly due to fragmented financing. As in the rest of the EU, financing for health and welfare services is currently under review. In 1990 financing for alarm systems came from the national health service, private medical insurance companies, social security, Government funds and contributions from patients. Lack of co-ordination was reported between institutional care and home care.

There are three forms of service provision:

- the subsidized sector

- the semi-commercial sector

- the commercial sector.

The subsidized sector is the most commonly found type of organization. It is run locally by social welfare offices for the elderly. Government subsidy has been reduced in recent years, which has motivated small offices to join together into larger regional organizations in order to get a more secure financial basis. Service subscription rates are low (about US $7 a month) and are paid by the user.

The semi-commercial sector is a new and growing area related to home care. The move to the community means services will be more client oriented and accessible. Centres are being established, staffed with qualified nurses. A range of other services may be offered. Demand for telemedical services is increasing. Home care services are better equipped to meet this need than traditional alarm organizations for the elderly. Furthermore, the activities of home care organizations are not limited to the elderly. Subscription charges are low in this sector too.

In The Netherlands, the commercial sector has always been active in the alarm services market. Subscription rates are about US $20–30 per month, paid by the user. Commercial organizations have no selection criteria for acceptance of clients.

Service provision

The Institute for Rehabilitation Research (IRV) at Hoensbroek is involved in a number of EC projects. During the time of the author's visit, an international FASDE project meeting was occurring. It was therefore possible to meet with people working on FASDE, to talk with them and to view working prototypes of electronic alarms. All rely on the operation of a 'trigger' device by the user.

Messages come to the central control centre via the telephone system when the system is triggered by the user. Nearly all organizations have a 24-hour attended post to receive the emergency calls. These are service centres. Most of them have a central incident room. Service centres are based in residential nursing homes, neighbourhood watch posts, hospitals, medical centres, community centres or the emergency services (police, fire or ambulance). Having a service centre gives the opportunity to take advantage of an important technological development: the speech link. The speech link makes it possible to differentiate between false alarms and real alarms and thus identify when a medical emergency exists.

In the long term, it is anticipated that the trigger will communicate with a standard home terminal which will be introduced by the telephone companies as a replacement for the telephone. These terminals will be able to send and receive integrated broadband communications (IBC): speech, video and other data.

Users

Evaluations of users' views and experiences are routinely performed by IRV. User satisfaction with the alarm system is reported as high. People apply for an alarm system and because they are self-selected, they have a positive attitude towards alarms.

Some housing projects for the elderly include alarm systems as standard provision. People moving into these homes need to take the system as a matter of course. The availability of a portable trigger (eg on a pendant) contributes to user satisfaction. However, evaluation in 1990 reported some criticisms:

- Inadvertent operation of the switch is possible.

- A portable trigger is an ugly thing to wear.

- Irritation of the neck may be caused by the cord.

If alarms are to be effective, they require user compliance. It has been found that there is resistance amongst a sizeable group of users to wearing the portable trigger all day. At least one third of users do not wear it when feeling well. In potentially dangerous situations (eg bathrooms and kitchens) the portable trigger may be out of reach. Freedom of choice about whether or not to wear the trigger must lead to some reduction in the effectiveness of the service.

It is interesting to note here a situation that occurred on a another case study visit, to Germany. The visit was in connection with the videotelephony (VT) project (*see* Chapter 7). When we visited a user at home, she was keen to show us how she used the VT equipment. During the visit, her pendant trigger lay on the sideboard. She said that she didn't like to wear it when she was feeling well.

People who have experienced a real alarm situation are reported as being generally satisfied with the way help was organized.

The future

The tendency is to integrate more alarm functions into the system (such as a smoke alarm, hypothermia alarm and medical devices). There is also a trend to integrate non-alarm functions in the system (such as auto dial functions for normal telephone calls, remote telephone answering via the trigger, and telephone amplifiers).

The EC FASDE contact person (all projects) was contacted about possible future developments. In his view:

'General trends are that electronic alarms are getting cheaper, so more accessible. Currently (1993) they cost around £200 each in the UK (where there has been more technical input), whereas in Germany they are still around £800. A unique feature of one of the current UK units is a 10-year battery which will reduce user anxiety and servicing costs. Triggers will also become more comfortable and less ugly.'

Review

The policy trend in The Netherlands is to promote care in the community, rather than in institutions. Provision of remote alarm services for the elderly and disabled supports this policy. Services offer most potential, and may be most cost effective when offered as part of an integrated care package. Fragmentation of service delivery systems and financing arrangements threaten the goal of integrated care.

Whilst alarm response systems seem to be valued by users, there remains a degree of resistance to wearing the remote trigger (pendant) throughout the course of daily life. This is a problem that needs to be overcome if the technology is to achieve its full potential. The FASDE team are well aware of this problem, and believe the solution to lie in the development of wrist-watch alarms. Not only will these be more comfortable to wear, they will be less stigmatizing for users.

Alarm systems: Canada

Like Europe, Canada has a 'greying' population. A major demographic shift was noted in 1986 when, for the first time, half of the population was found to be over 31 years of age. This trend, together with a concomitant fall in the birth rate, was reported in a Government 'Futures' document aimed at predicting health needs in the year 2000 and beyond (IHCFF, 1988). These trends are also referred to in *The Rainbow Report*, a report of the Premiers Commission on future health care for Albertans, (Premiers Commission, 1989). This was a major exercise in participatory democracy in health care choices, organized by the Alberta Government at the end of the 1980s. It offered opportunities for all Albertans to influence the direction of future health care policy. Participation was made possible by use of electronic town hall (ETH) technology (referred to in Chapter 8).

A *Rainbow Report* finding was that people wished to have control of their lives, and to live in their homes and communities, with support, for as long as they were able. As in Europe, a way to meet this need is by provision of alarm support services.

Service description

The alarm support service studied is offered through LIFELINE. LIFELINE is a commercial organization based in Massachusetts, USA. It provides personal response systems (PRS) and monitoring services throughout the USA and Canada. PRS are devices connected to a user's telephone that, when activated, send a 'help' signal to a monitoring centre. LIFELINE provides PRS and other services to people with health limitations, physical challenges or personal security needs.

The communicator unit is the voice communicator that links individuals living independently at home to care professionals. The unit is a small table-top device, about the size of a textbook stood on its end. The unit transmits an electronic message via the telephone line to alert the response centre that help may be needed. When the response centre receives the signal, the subscriber is called to provide assurance over the built-in speaker phone, and assistance if needed. The unit is activated by pressing the pendant or unit personal help button. Automatic two-way voice transmission permits immediate communication between the user and the response centre. The built-in speaker phone also allows users to answer routine telephone calls without having to get to the phone.

Other features include:

- a rechargeable battery
- a reset message feature (to indicate that help has arrived)
- a 'help still needed' feature (to indicate that help has not yet arrived)
- periodic telephone and powerline checks. (The telephone line is checked every four hours)
- warning indicator lights which warn the user of a line failure, equipment fault or emergency battery use.

In Edmonton, LIFELINE services are offered by the Good Samaritan Society (a Lutheran social services organization). This is a non-profit making organization begun in 1949. Membership is made up of both Lutherans and non-Lutherans whose main objective is to provide services to the elderly, the handicapped and the disadvantaged.

LIFELINE serves the Greater Edmonton area and provides 24-hour cover for five communities in northern Alberta. Funding for the society's operations comes primarily from Government grants. Clients and residents contribute about 22% of the funds. The control mechanism and the 24-hour service cost much more than the monthly $25 charge to the elderly and disabled people who have pendants. Nevertheless, if the charge is more than a person can afford, the society offers subsidies.

A volunteer program is maintained in which over 500 volunteers are registered, most of whom are active on a regular basis. LIFELINE monitors close to 1000 users through two computer data consoles. Trained professional staff are available 24 hours a day, every day. According to the service manager:

> 'LIFELINE is the Good Samaritans' extension into the community. We offer extensive support to our users through a social support network and volunteer programme. To this point, we strive to ensure that our programme is more than just electronic equipment. We view the LIFELINE units as the entry point into the community support programme.'

An audit by LIFELINE systems (Massachusetts) of the 10 largest programmes in North America (January 1992) placed the Edmonton Good Samaritan LIFELINE service first, with an average response time of 27 seconds. The response time was measured from the moment of pushing the personal help pendant to the time the monitor's voice was heard asking what type of help was required.

Users

Data are available on the 463 Edmonton users (January 1993). The user profile gives five most common primary medical diagnoses in descending order:

- stroke

- hypertension

- diabetes

- cancer

- multiple sclerosis.

Interestingly, in addition to elderly and disabled people, the alarm service is offered to the parents of premature infants, who are provided with a unit when the infant is discharged from hospital.

Distribution of users by language of origin is:

- English   396

- French   17

- German   15

- Ukranian   9

- Dutch   4

- Polish   4

- Chinese   4

Fourteen language groups in all are represented. Efforts are made to meet the language need of all groups. Surprisingly, only one member of the Inuit population (Cree Indian) is represented. This could, however, reflect different cultural value systems and care networks, rather than inequity. Nonetheless, it is a source of concern to staff, who want to ensure that support is available to all who need it.

Data are also held on emergencies attended. In February 1993 (Greater Edmonton and other areas: 1000 users) 129 emergencies were responded to. Most (37%) were in both instances in the 56–60 year age group. It is interesting to note that only 24% were in the 76-years-old and over category.

Ninety-three percent of users were living alone at time of the emergency. Reasons for calling (by primary medical diagnosis) were related to:

	%
• multiple sclerosis	47
• cerebrovascular disease	14.29
• cerebal palsy	12

The following extracts are typical of user responses accrued by both telephone interview and letters to LIFELINE:

'I was awakened by severe pains in the stomach. LIFELINE notified an ambulance . . . it arrived in record time and transferred me to the hospital where it found that my ulcer was active again. After prescribing medication, the doctor released me. The prompt help saved me from pain and other consequences. I'm doing nicely at home now on the medication.' (middle-aged female user)

When returning equipment following recovery from a period of illness, one subscriber wrote:

'It has been a pleasure being associated with you. I felt I had many friends. All of you were always courteous and pleasant to talk to. That part I will miss. Wishing you all the best.' (elderly male user)

One user's story is particularly illustrative of the independence experienced by two supported older people:

'Dear good friends,
   The following is to request my LIFELINE service to be discontinued in the one-month notice period. I would like to thank all the people behind your wonderful organization for the service and feeling of great security it has given me. I am not discontinuing it because of cost or dissatisfaction. My wife and I are going south for a little sun and upon our return may move into a condo and let someone else do the shovelling and mowing. At that time, the good Lord willing, I'll resume the service if I'm permitted. In the meantime, others more in need can use the monitor and pendant. When I began LIFELINE, I was in recovery from major heart surgery and my wife had to fly east to be with her terminally ill parents. LIFELINE became my dependable emergency partner at night and when I was alone. I cannot praise too much the people with whom I came into contact . . . who sometimes had to put up with a forgetful old geezer. If you can send me a pledge card or some such, I would like to make a contribution in the coming year . . .' (middle-aged male user)

The goal of Good Samaritan staff is to seek to maintain the high standards they have already achieved. Whilst they currently feel comfortable about their ability to do this, they are concerned about the possibility of grant cuts as Alberta, like the rest of Canada and Europe, is in economic recession.

Review

The service is a demonstrable model of good practice. It serves a recognized community need highly efficiently and sensitively. Currently it is available to all Albertans who need it. A particularly imaginative use is in neonatal support, enabling infants to be cared for by their parents in the community, thus helping to meet the twin health policy goals of care in the community and cost efficiency. Parents also have the reassurance that emergency services are quickly available, should they be needed.

Summary of alarm systems

Quality

Indications are that alarm systems are a high quality service, and are generally valued by users. Some users do not like the current form of provision (trigger pendant), so do not wear it when they are feeling well. As accidents are, by definition, unplanned, they happen to 'well' people. The nature of some diseases and disabilities is also unpredictable. That some users fail to achieve 24-hour cover must be a cause for concern. Technological developments are now occurring, however, which mean that product acceptability should increase with the introduction of prototype wrist-watches.

Skills and teamworking

Evidence of appropriate use of professional skills and collaborative teamworking were found in both the FASDE and the LIFELINE schemes. LIFELINE, however, seems better able to withstand fragmentation of services as it is so closely integrated into both local community support systems and local consciousness. This may of course be true of user services in the other FASDE countries, but the view in The Netherlands was that there was not cohesive service coverage.

Cost

Both Canada and The Netherlands have social security systems available to support aids for personal living, so the cost to the consumer may be small or non-existent. In both countries, of course, consumers are free to purchase equipment direct from manufacturers if they so wish. Indications are that the costs of these may differ markedly between individual countries.

As with other preventive health promotion schemes, costs to government are difficult to establish. However, as with the domiciliary fetal monitoring scheme (Chapter 3), it may be assumed that out-patient community support costs will be less than in-patient care or full institutional support (ie nursing home costs).

Equity

Alarm systems are a relatively cheap and effective aid to support independent living. They have two main benefits. Firstly they give a feeling of safety to individuals, and secondly they make organization of adequate help possible at (usually rare) times of emergency. They can support independent living in all types of individuals and families, from premature babies through to the frail elderly.

Use of medical technology means that more infants become viable and more people can live longer. Alarm systems offer user friendly low technology support for independent living in the community.

Social integration

A paper by IRV (1990) cites a number of evaluation studies which show that the frequency of social visits to elderly people (family, friends and neighbours) does not decrease when an alarm system is installed. People who pay visits are freed from the monitoring task and their visit then becomes a social call.

There are sound economic and social reasons for supporting frail elderly people to live at home, rather than institutionalizing them. Morally and ethically, this strategy is also to be commended. Elderly citizens should be able to live independently, with dignity, and know that emergency services can be summoned should they be needed.

7 Telehealth and Social Support

'. . . since I am connected, I am much more organized . . .'

(user)

Type of service

Social support.

Technology

Videotelephony using a copper coaxial cable system (Germany), and a fibre optic system (Portugal). Details of how each system operates are given in the text relating to each country.

The videotelephony (VT) project is part of the RACE programme: 1054: Application Pilot for People with Special Needs (APPSN). The RACE (Research and Development in Advanced Communication Technologies in Europe) objectives are to make a major contribution towards the implementation of integrated broadband communications (IBC) in Europe and to contribute to regional development within the community, by allowing less developed regions to benefit fully from telecommunications developments (project line 7: Advanced Communication Experiments).

Location

To help with selection of case study visits, the author met with the APPSN project evaluator and reviewed the stages and characteristics of all the EC VT pilots. Aveiro in Portugal was said to be a demonstrator project taking an interesting approach in a poor country. The pilot in Frankfurt, Germany, was described as a large project, focusing on the elderly and using cable TV networks. Visits to both these pilots were advised, and were consequently undertaken.

Population

Elderly and disabled people.

Context

In the EU, the population of elderly people will total 56 million by the year 2000 and the disabled will total 36–48 million (Organization for Economic Co-operation and Development, 1988). The changing demographic structure of Europe means that support of the elderly and those with special needs is a major policy issue for health care providers. In particular, the need for social services is growing. Currently this need is realized through regular domiciliary visits, 'sheltered' housing schemes and residential (institutional) care. All the evidence to date suggests that this latter option is the one least preferred by service users.

The videotelephony pilots trial support services for the elderly and disabled, and demonstrate to RACE the types of support services in the care sector that will be commercially viable using videotelephony.

During his meeting with the author, the evaluator commented that the RACE pilots were currently highly technical; social issues had hardly been addressed, but would be tackled in the next RACE project, 20/23, on telecommunity:

> 'It's mainly technologists and psychologists with an experimental bent; we don't have social workers or people who have cared for the elderly over a long period of time and have a feel for the issues. It's a bit early yet. We're used to managers talking to managers . . .'

In its origins, the RACE project has some similarities to HANDYNET, which was also, initially, technologically and commercially led. As will be seen from the case study data, however, RACE is much more user receptive.

Videotelephony: Germany

The Frankfurt pilot is one of the RACE APPSN pilots. Technical work is being led by Alcatel-SEL, who are also managing the internal consortium. The organizing institution in Frankfurt is Empirica GmbH, which is also the lead organization for the German part of the next phase of RACE, on telecommunity, which is ongoing.

Visits were made to two care institutions, one of which includes the service centre, and the homes of two users in Rodelheim, the project setting.

In the Frankfurt pilot, Empirica-Tekom (Bonn) has the role of co-ordinating the development of services, managing them, and carrying out an evaluation of the APPSN pilot. Work is done in co-operation with the Nassauisches Heim Siedlungsbaugesellschaft, the major provider of housing for lower income groups in Frankfurt. The services in the pilot are run by the Frankfurter Verband fur Alten-und Behindertenhilfe e. V, a care organization providing the majority of sheltered housing and old people's homes and day centres in Frankfurt am Main. It also provides alarm telephony services to over a thousand clients in the area. Funding for staffing the pilot service has been provided by the City of Frankfurt. The VT pilot project offers 17 clients (15 households) videotelephony services.

The videotelephony services on trial have the overall aim of promoting the ability of the elderly and mobility impaired to live independently, and to reduce the load on social service resources.

Service description

Services are provided to some residents in sheltered apartments adjacent to the service centre setting, and to some residents living on a large housing estate in the community. The housing estate in which the pilot VT service is installed is interesting because it was built in the late 1920s as part of the international 'garden cities' movement. Ernst May was the architect. At a time of recession, mass unemployment and housing shortages, May decided to build a garden colony for socially disadvantaged families. Today the estate houses around 25 000 people, mainly with low incomes. The high percentage of elderly people was a major reason for selecting the estate as the site of the Frankfurt pilot. In parallel with early service development, a needs assessment survey with potential users was carried out, and users' views were built into design solutions.

The service centre for the videotelephony is located in the afore-mentioned care institution. Clients are connected to the service centre by a network based on copper coaxial cables. Cable was said to have been chosen for the superiority of its picture quality. In addition to transmissions from the centre, two reverse channels are used to pass pictures captured by the camera in the clients' homes back to the service centre. Special terminal equipment has been developed, consisting of a television set modified to enable both normal TV viewing and interactive audiovisual communication to the service centre. A camera mounted above the TV has a moderatively wide field of view, normally showing a client in the preferred position for TV viewing. A shutter can be easily moved in front of the camera by clients who do not trust the electronic system to protect them from being seen. The casing below the monitor houses the equipment to enable the set to transmit camera pictures back through the network. An integrated microphone provides quality of sound similar to that of normal TV. A simplified remote control device was specially developed to make operation as easy as possible. Care has been taken to position equipment so that there is a good view of both the adviser's and the user's face. Maintenance of eye contact is considered particularly important.

Services are provided from a room located in the care centre. This room has a service desk integrating the monitor/camera combination for VT, a PC with monitor, a document camera and a video recorder. The PC software is a DOS application. Terminal equipment is managed by a small team of professionally trained staff. Working in single person shifts, two women and one man provide support six hours per day.

The residential centre

Frankfurter Verband fur Alten-und Behindertenhilfe e. V (FV) is a residential and day-care centre for local elderly people who need support. There are two types of resident: those needing continuing care and support, and those needing minimal care. Continuing care residents are either physically or mentally frail (for example, 60% are clinically 'confused'). These 144 residents are cared for by a multidisciplinary team of staff including social workers, nurses, a physiotherapist, a gymnastic teacher and an occupational therapist. They receive medical care from their own family doctor.

In addition to care beds, there are 42 sheltered apartments for older people. Three nurses help residents with activities of daily living that they are unable to manage for themselves. These residents, as well as members of the local community, are able to use all of the support services offered by the centre, from chiropody to swimming and hairdressing. Strong efforts are made to integrate the centre into the life of the local community. Special days are celebrated by public events, such as a band concert on Mother's Day. 'Tea dances' are held on Friday afternoons, which in addition to residents, are attended by between 40 and 50 local older people.

According to the centre manager, the goal is

'to integrate the town into the house, and to bring our people outside'.

This process is facilitated by the provision of a cafeteria, where residents and non-residents can mingle socially. As all residents are local, they are able to maintain their friendships and social contacts. The cafeteria is run by three residents, who each receive 150 DM per week for four hours' work a day.

Local integration of both the centre and the VT service (operated by the centre) is considered important with regard to their future use. Personal relationships can be developed and maintained, even though the nature and degree of health care and social support may change over time.

Once a link between the client and the service centre has been made, the client can be provided with assistance. Service components are:

- active information and care for elderly people living alone

- remote response to emergencies (anxious clients can receive help and reassurance as and when they need it)

- information and assistance (using the document camera, clients can be helped to fill out/understand complex forms and bills)

- support for therapy/physiotherapy (live and videotaped 'refresher' sessions are offered)

- remote access to expertise (experts can be brought in to answer questions direct to clients)

- support for carers (carers can be given relief from their 24-hour job by a 'remote' care service).

The remote care service is the one which is most ethically controversial. To avoid misuse:

- contractually, both patient and carer have to agree its use

- the client can, at any time, cancel remote care calls by using a switch on their home equipment.

Users

Evaluation of services occurred in 1992, from January to December. At the beginning, the call average was 10 per day; towards the end of the year, the average rose to 11 per day. A sizeable minority of calls (39%) lasted less than five minutes. Sixteen per cent of calls lasted between five and 10 minutes and 22% between 15 and 30 minutes. In 9% of all cases, contact between client and service centre was established for longer than half an hour.

Most of the elderly users had no problems in using the equipment. In general, the service was rated very positively. Suggestions for improvements concerned additional personnel and longer service hours. Almost all of the users emphasized the very personal and close relationship to staff. Five believe it directly changed their lives. Statements collected ranged from 'I don't feel lonely anymore' to 'I have a more regular daily routine, I have regular meals again' and 'I have more joy in my life'. Two users were visited in their homes by the author – see Figure 11.

Frau **A** is a widowed lady in her late eighties. She has limited mobility, and is thus largely housebound. She is in receipt of no other social services. Her home is alive with drawings, a hobby which she has just begun in the last two years. Frau **A** also has an alarm pendant. She is enthusiastic about both the VT and alarm services, as she believes they allow her to stay safe and in control of her own life in the home she has lived in for over 60 years. Her 'best thing' about the technology is the freedom it gives her to live her life as she wishes.

Frau **B** is a widowed lady, also in her eighties. Unlike Frau **A**, Frau **B** has no physical limitations. Recently Frau **B** became involved again with the 'Grey Panthers' organization (she was active before her husband's death).

About the service she says, 'When my husband died I lost all interest. The service got me involved in life again'. Owing to severe depression caused by grieving, Frau **B** was invited by the counselling service to take part in the Frankfurt pilot. That was two and a half years ago. Now, each morning, she participates in the transmitted gymnastic session, then calls in for a few words with the adviser. Her 'best thing' about the service is the social contact it offers. When asked what she used the service for (information, advice, care, etc) she looked slightly puzzled and replied, 'Why, to talk to Frau **X**' (the service provider). For Frau **B** the service benefit was a decrease in her social isolation by providing a hook back into the outside world.

Figure 11:   Profiles of two videotelephony users

Discussions with project staff and service centre staff showed they recognized the demographic shifts that are occurring in Germany and elsewhere

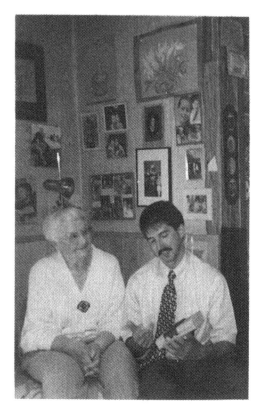

Figure 12: A demonstration of videotelephony

in Europe, the need to fund care from insurance systems, and the need to make 'best choices' in health care.

Currently there is a debate in Germany on how health care systems will be introduced. It is predicted (Robinson, 1992) that when an insurance system is introduced it will lead to a considerable expansion of care services. Within the context of this debate, it is believed that videotelephony can be a valuable, cost-effective form of social and health support for elderly people. Moreover, research by Erkert (Erkert, 1992; Erkert et al., 1993) has shown that videotelephony could be a very acceptable means of supplying support services.

As part of the APPSN pilot, Erkert made a study of the social networks of the elderly. Fifty-three people living in a housing estate with a dispropor-tionate number of elderly residents were interviewed. It was found that many of these elderly did not have an extensive communication network. The most important contacts were face-to-face contacts, and the most important social network, the family. High telephone and television usage was found and it is hypothesized that the lonely elderly form pseudo-relationships with television personalities in order to fill their social contact needs. This 'hook' can be used to provide a new form of social contact (videotelephony) for the elderly, using technologies with which they are already familiar.

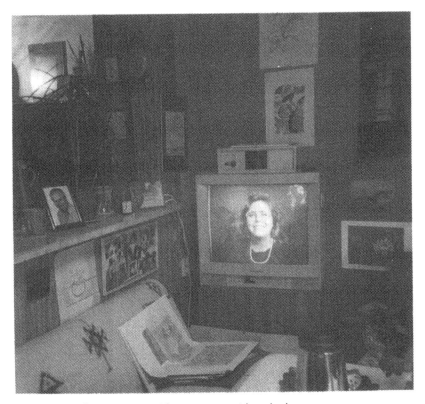

Figure 13:   The service provider seen on a videotelephone screen

However, it was strongly expressed during the visit to the pilot site that videotelephony is only one of a range of care services that may be offered (as is residential care or home visiting). The most appropriate support service will be determined by both client need and client wishes. Videotelephony, if it is to fulfil its potential, should be part of an integrated care and support network.

The future

In the future it is believed that there will be further development of ambulatory care and self care, using the new technologies.

Future plans for the Frankfurt pilot are:

* to connect users to each other, as well as to the service centre.

   The next centre to be connected, Auguste Oberwinter Haus, was also visited. This is a residential centre for young and middle-aged disabled people. Flats containing basic equipment are provided and residents encouraged to have their own furniture and decorations. The theme of local integration is very evident; some residents work at the reception, others run the lively cafeteria. The plan is to provide VT services as part of the telecommunity pilot.

- to continue work on RACE telecommunity (1992–94). The goal is to extend videotelephony support services to various forms of sheltered accommodation, including that for disabled people.

- technical changes, including provision of client to client communication, and making a gateway into the ISDN network

- to offer more multidisciplinary technical training. (Technical training was given at the beginning of the project and staff were chosen from multi-disciplinary care backgrounds.)

Review

The Frankfurt pilot is an excellent model of good practice in provision of support services to elderly people. Prior to service provision, a needs analysis was carried out with the target population to inform decisions about service provision. There is evidence of listening to and involving users at all stages of this pilot, and of sensitivity to, and best use of local social life. The thorough, extensive and sensitive groundwork that has occurred in the APPSN pilot should prove a sound base from which to develop the new RACE pilot on telecommunity.

Videotelephony: Portugal

Unlike Germany, Portugal is regarded as one of the poorer EU countries. Both its telecommunications and primary health care services are evolving with, as yet, fairly limited infrastructures. With regard to telecommunications, however, Portugal is benefiting from funding and positive discrimination in terms of EC research activity.

The setting for the RACE VT pilot in Portugal is the Centro de Estudos de Telecomunicacoes (CET). The centre is involved in a number of RACE projects. In addition to the Application Pilot for People with Special Needs (APPSN), it is operating on Better Infrastructure for Rural Development (BIRD).

The APPSN Portugese pilot allows the provision of remote support services to elderly people in their homes by use of videotelephony. Videotelephony provision is by a 2 Mbps circuit switched network, using fibre optic cables. At the time of visiting (December 1992) the capacity for VT services was for 28 users homes. For demonstration purposes, six homes were used. VT visits were made to these homes. Transmission (image) quality was very high, but staff believed that this may act as a limitation, as it is very expensive. Different capacities were generated and viewed and it was suggested that it would be possible to use 384 kbs, which is less expensive, not demonstrably inferior, and can support 140 users.

In addition to communications between users and the service centre, users can call up each other.

In discussions with the APPSN team, the following points were made:

- The **cost** of VT can appear high because the infrastructure to support it needs to be developed. In this case, it is the ISDN system, expected in Portugal within 10 years.

- The '**added value**' can be high. Service providers (doctors, priests, social workers and educators) can visit homes by VT, thus saving the cost of physical home visits. The main benefit, however, is seen as supporting people at home, where they prefer to be.

- Another advantage is that VT can produce integrated, more cost-effective services, although politicians and planners still need to be convinced to invest in it. This entails **revaluing the elderly** and their place in society: they need to be seen as valued contributing members, rather than simply a drain on resources.

Service description

The service centre (through which communications are routed) is a welfare institution providing both day and residential services to the elderly. The services provided are:

- social and medical advice and information
- religious services
- gymnastics classes
- 24-hour 'hotline' support for users' queries.

The manager of the service centre was enthusiastic about the pilot, although there were problems – not with the service itself, but with support. For example, the doctor consulted is the service centre doctor and not the family physician and this can sometimes lead to problems. Moreover, there are no nurses attached to communicate with or to make domiciliary visits. This is partly due to the fact that primary care is very new in Portugal (since 1986) and also that a family doctor may have his own nurse.

When asked which of the services people used most and seemed to value most, the reply was social services and gymnastics. In this instance, social services should be seen as information. The week the author visited, there was a Christmas party and users were very excited about this, mentioning it spontaneously, and all planning to go.

Users

Data held by CET show that the system is easy to use and is liked by users, and observations and interviews support this view. Four VT visits were made and visits were made to two homes. In both instances, both partners were ambulatory; they were not housebound and were not hearing or visually impaired. All were in their mid-seventies.

The first couple were middle-class living in a large house. The VT unit was in the living room. The unit is big (about the size of an American type refrigerator), but did not dominate the room. The wife likes the service to check on medical advice with the service centre, the husband for social contact with his friend. He was competent and confident with the equipment and there was obvious pleasure in making the communication. He was very keen to tell me about the last party he went to at the service centre (previous to being involved in the VT pilot neither had used the centre). At the party he met an old school friend he had not seen for 60 years. He was so excited that when he returned home he called up CET to tell them.

The second couple were working-class, living in a very small house. The unit dominated the small living room which was shared by husband, wife, daughter and grandchild. None the less they appeared enthusiastic about the VT. When asked which service they preferred (videotelephony or telephone: both were present), they immediately and enthusiastically replied 'videotelephony', as had the previous couple. For them the image was very important:

> 'You can see your friends. I wish our daughter in France had one. It would be wonderful to see her and see how she is.'

Although the wife mentioned the value of medical advice from the service centre, the couple saw the major value of VT as its social function:

> 'I don't know what it will be like when they take it away.'

The future

Pilot staff believed that, in the future, the APPSN project will benefit work on the BIRD project. It is planned that VT will be used to provide telelibrary, telelearning and telecounter services. It is considered very important that the elderly be seen as valued members of society. The plan is to have elderly people pass on Portuguese traditions, customs and folk art to schoolchildren by teleteaching. This form of remote cross generational communication is one that offers exciting potential for youngsters, older citizens, and communities. It is explored in some detail in Chapter 8, as part of the Reading citizen's TV initiative.

Review

There seems little doubt that the system is valued by these users. Observations confirmed that the system is easy to use, and gives both information and pleasure in use. It has also created new social networks that did not previously exist, and use of services previously unknown.

Summary of videotelephony

Quality

With regard to meeting both social and (some) medical needs, the provision of VT support services seem ideally suited to some groups of citizens, namely the frail elderly and disabled. Evidence of demonstrable good practice existed in both the pilots visited. The technology was found to be well accepted, highly valued and easy to use. Indeed the indications are that, in this instance, the market is ready, waiting and even impatient for provision:

'It *is* the future for some people, so far as we see it. We're seeing that in the evaluation. Because some people want to live in their own home. They don't want to live in care. They want to live in their own home, but they don't want to be alone. They're frightened . . . they hear about old ladies falling down and not getting up . . . the likelihood is small but the outcome is quite dire, so they're afraid. There are reports from social workers, in Germany for example, that with VT people become mobilized again and reactivated . . . because they're building relationships with people they can see, whereas they won't build relationships with people they can only hear. There was an old lady whose husband died. She went into withdrawal . . . they selected her as a candidate . . . she's not very communicative. Her old man was very quiet, but they had this ritual. When he came home he washed, he made the coffee and they sat and talked about the day . . . she talked about the garden . . . and that was her hook into the world . . . without that she was lost. And so now daily she makes her call to the service centre at 5 o'clock, the service provider gets her coffee ready, they have a chat and she's back on her feet again, for the sake of five or 10 minutes a day. It's stories like that give you heart . . . we don't have enough expertise on the project of that type.' (evaluator).

Cost

Costs were viewed as low by the APPSN evaluator:

'You can buy a VT for £400. Then there's rental and call charges. you could be looking at a system for less than £1000 within five years. The cost is very low compared to the alternatives. If you imagine, a deaf association has to train and house interpreters, they spend 50–70% of their time in the traffic, for example going to a doctor's surgery or a court to act for the deaf person, all that commuting time is wasted. These old people in Germany can ring up the service provider with queries "tell me what I should do . . ." It's very short and it's very immediate. To send workers out into the field costs a lot of money, they should be doing what they're good at. Also housing people in residential care is very expensive . . . if you can enable someone to stay in their own home by providing them with a few thousand pounds of electrical equipment, it's got to be better.'

Teamwork

A well planned and delivered VT service increases the potential for team-working. Better use can be made of the professional skills of different care team members, and service provision can be maximized, in that services that are offered in care settings that are also VT service centres can be transmitted (live or on videotape) to the broader user audience in the community. This makes the service more equitable and more cost-effective.

Social integration

Videotelephony has the potential to extend social networks for the house-bound. It also has the potential to form an electronic substitute for face-to-face visiting and provision of remote care services. Like the other telehealth innovations discussed in this text, however, telematics needs to be understood as part of a total care package, not a substitute for it. Having said this, as we shall see in Chapter 8, old age does not necessarily mean dependence. For the vast majority of Europeans, properly organized social support to promote independent living will allow for minimal, rather than major, state dependency.

8 Telehealth and Public Policy

'. . . giving the "shut-ins" a say'

(service provider)

Whilst the focus of this book has been an exploration of the use of telematic services in health promotion and medical care, another major concern is public participation in health care decision making. In discussions with a number of experts, prior to choice of case studies, two North American innovations were repeatedly mentioned as examples of good practice in electronic public participation in decision making. These were the electronic town meeting (ETM) concept, and the Reading citizen's TV project. Both were visited.

Electronic town meetings: Canada

Type of service

Public participation in policy formulation.

Technology

Electronic town meetings (ETMs). ETMs permit simultaneous dialogue between large numbers of people in different locations. They work by combining a live television broadcast with feedback from a pre-selected scientific sample of citizens. A moderator, a panel and a studio audience discuss a pressing community issue in a live television broadcast. As the discussion develops and important questions become apparent, the moderator addresses them to the random sample in the viewing audience. The viewers cast their votes on the questions by dialling 1–800 numbers on their telephones.

Location

Edmonton, Canada.

Population

People who are housebound or unable to attend public meetings.

Context

Visionaries such as Buckminster Fuller, Erich Fromm, Hazel Henderson and Amitai Etzioni have foreseen the potential of informatics in promoting electronic democracy. One vehicle for electronic democracy is electronic town meetings.

Since 1970, there have been many experiments in both Canada and the US with electronic democracy. Frequently these were low profile 'one off' types of events. This changed in 1992–93 when use of ETMs in the USA presidential campaign put them on the public agenda. Throughout North America (USA and Canada) there is now great interest in their use. In 1990, in Alberta, Canada, ETMs were used to involve citizens in helping formulate Government health policies for the future.

Service description

Facing the Future Inc., working in partnership with ACCESS network (a local cable TV company), and the Edmonton Board of Health presented the first electronic town meeting to Canada on 3rd April 1990. The programme explored the reactions of the citizens of Edmonton to the prevention and promotion recommendations of the Premier's Commission of future health care for Albertans (see page 85, Chapter 6).

How the system works, and the case of *Rainbow report* participation was described by the Director of Facing the Future Inc., (**M**):

'It's a combination of broadcast or cable TV and computerized telephone voting, allied with voice messaging. You use a televized focus group . . . typically what you have is a moderator, a panel, a studio audience that interact around an issue . . . like Oprah Winfrey; a chat show format . . . around serious issues, where you want to map out what the issues are, how people perceive them. Or it can be used as means by which you can achieve consensus. It works by a presentation (five to seven minutes of video/head and shoulders talk, charts) then the panel talk about it, then you get an interaction with the audience going.

The audience is chosen according to whatever criterion you want by networking, ahead of time. You assemble a random sample in the community. You send out to people a set of phone numbers that enable them to vote (these are confidential). When they dial they are automatically hooked up to a call counting computer in the telephone system. The count gets automatically translated by a modem to a computer in the studio and within three to five minutes you have the result.

The random sample is there so you get a good accurate reading of what the general public response is, to whatever the issue is. Additional things that can be done, you can also bring in qualitative comments; you can give people 1–800 (toll free) numbers to call in and give opinions.'

Costs were then discussed which, surprisingly, were low:

'As part of the licensing agreement companies have to provide Canada Community Cable (CCC) channel free of charge to anybody who qualifies as a community group under the definition of the Canadian Radio and Television Commission (CRTC). So if you use that you have zero broadcasting costs, the actual call counting for a city the size of Edmonton (needing a sample of 450 people) costs less than $1000. The phone company charges for each call that goes into the computer (usually 50 cents), and on top of that they make a set up charge . . . about $250. So six questions, 450 people voting, 50 cents a time, plus the $250 works out at somewhere between $600 and $1000.'

With any innovation there is a need for visionary people to recognize and maximize opportunity when it occurs. This is what **M** did:

'The Minister of (Social) Affairs in this province was interested in getting people's ideas on health . . . I had some inside contacts (at the Board of Health) . . . I knew about his work in participatory democracy and futures work in general, so I asked to talk to him about ways to increase public participation . . .
   We set up town hall meetings in about 300 communities throughout the province, each of them addressing what should be the desired future of the community. We ran an ETH pilot around the health promotion recommendations of the previous Commission. The Board of Health and the Commission put up about $5000. I persuaded ACCESS to give studio time free, another (friend) got phone time for nothing. So the whole thing was done for less than $4000. The Commission was there as a panel (in the studio) with an audience of interested people (from Edmonton). We broadcast to the whole province and also used 1–800 lines for additional qualitative inputs.'

We went on to talk about equity in participation:

'Your usual town meeting only brings out those with an axe to grind, so you don't hear from the general public, the "shut-ins", the immobile, the socially disadvantaged; those groups don't get reached by a regular town hall, or any hearings process as usually practised in "democracies". ETHs reach all those people. As long as you have a phone or TV (98% of Edmonton's population), you can participate.'

Review

ETMs, set up and used correctly, have the potential to influence public policy for the greater good of citizens. For ETMs to be efficiently and effectively utilized, however, there needs to be both an adequate telecommunications infrastructure in place and a participatory style of government which encourages citizens to believe that their concerns will be acknowledged.

Community television: USA

Type of service

Promotion of community participation by interactive community television.

Technology

Cable television. Originally equipment was crude and heavy, and offered black and white pictures only. In the 1980s advances in cable technology made it more effective and accessible. Colour video equipment became available at reasonable cost, with greatly enhanced performance. At this time the system was built to its current 61 channel capacity. This receives signals from satellites, microwave and over-the-air broadcasts. Berks Cable Company processes and amplifies these signals and delivers them to homes in a 700 mile radius. The monthly cost is stated as 'less than taking your family to see just one movie at the theatre' (producer).

Location

Berks, Reading, in Pennsylvania.

Population

All citizens in the reception area.

Context

Like Canadians, Americans have a very strong sense of their right to shape the communities that they live in. They are also more comfortable with technology than Europeans. However, the USA has a free market economy which not only thrives on, but actively promotes competition in all spheres of public life. As in other Western countries, wealth and progress are defined in purely economic terms, and as in Europe, there have been growing signs of unease with this approach. According to Henderson (1993), now is the time to redefine wealth and progress:

'We need to throw out the old Cold War, left/right, economic text books which are still used in colleges all over this country and in Europe, and we need to see the world anew, we need to reframe all those debates we see on TV and in the newspaper headlines that lead us to believe that free markets have triumphed, free trade is always good for everyone, global competitiveness is the new goal everywhere, economic efficiency is the top priority, citizens are now customers, democracy is equated with markets, budgets must be balanced, deficits are out of control, so cuts in jobs must be inevitable and the GNP must continue to grow.' (transcript, keynote address)

Henderson goes on to argue that the GNP of a country is only one (largely inappropriate), indicator of progress, and that many indicators, including qualitative ones, are necessary. In her view, the future direction for societies should be collaborative, multidisciplinary and sustainable. She urges the development of a global civic culture, underpinned by global citizens' television.

Service description

Cable television services are principally concerned with delivering mass entertainment to audiences in homes and communities. Local cable programming is unique because it is created by the people of each community, and reflects that area's distinct character and diversity. The mayor of Reading recognized this when planning permission for installing cable TV was sought in the 1960s; he agreed to it on the condition that some channels would be dedicated to community use. These became Berks Community TV (BCTV).

BCTV is provided by Berks Cable TV. It is a non-profit making organization. Their philosophy is:

'to improve the quality of life for the people of Reading and Berks county by encouraging dialogue among diverse segments of the community on a variety of topics. Through live interactive programmes produced by volunteers, BCTV brings to the community the best possible educational and informational programmes, and provides a unique opportunity for volunteer activities.' (Mission Statement)

BCTV began in the mid 1960s. In 1971 a mobile video production truck was constructed and public access workshops were offered. In 1975, the National Science Foundation awarded a grant to a consortium involving Berks Cable TV, New York University, the City of Reading and the Berks Senior Citizen's Council, to deliver social services to the elderly, using interactive cable TV. The following year this experimental programming was made available to all Berks cable TV subscribers.

Four channels are set aside for local programming, one each for:

- community access

- education access

- municipal access (town hall meetings)

- local events/interests.

Over 20 programme areas are offered. These include:

- Policing Reading, a bimonthly programme produced by the Bureau of Police. The topics highlighted in 1992 were crime prevention, substance abuse, and an introduction to the new Chief and Deputy Chief of Police.

- Bureau of Recreation, a monthly programme sponsored by the Bureau, that follows the recreation calendar from playgrounds to indoor activities at local recreation centres.

- Working for a Greater Reading, hosted by the executive assistant to the mayor and featuring people and events that enhance the city's living and working environment. 'The Reading Phillies', 'The City Greenhouse', 'Opening Penn Square' and 'Traffic Engineering' were some of the subjects for 1992.

- Reading Recycles, produced by the Bureau of Solid Waste, which is a monthly programme that updates on the city's recycling efforts.

- Hispanic Centre Presents, a Spanish language programme about the services and programmes available at the Hispanic Centre.

- Profiles on Development, hosted by the programme co-ordinator for community development. It features projects that receive money from the city's community development office. Facade improvement, the enterprise zone, and social service agencies are a few of the topics that were profiled in 1992.

- Televized Meetings, showing city council meetings: there were 54 council meetings televized live in 1992 from the council chambers in City Hall.

- Bridging the Generation Gap, a weekly programme in which high schools participate. This is hosted by former Reading mayor, Eugene L Shirk, who is now President of BCTV. Using two-way TV technology, students participate in this programme from their school studios or from a remote location in the area. Students choose a topic each week, research it, and go on 'live' with Mr Shirk. Senior citizens also participate in the pro-gramme, at the studio or from their homes by telephone. The unique concept of this programme, ie of providing a medium for senior citizens and young people to explore how and what others think, was the subject of a segment on the Learning Channel (national TV) in 1985, cited as an example of 'excellence in education'.

Users

As can be seen from the above description, users are both heavily involved in, and served by, BCTV. According to one of the original partners:

> 'the stars of local TV programming are not the actors and news anchors of traditional television, but instead are average citizens from all walks of life.'

In addition, C-SPAN 1 and 2 are offered. These are a public service of the cable TV industry, offering 'commercial free' live coverage of the US House of Representatives and Senate floor activity, plus other public events from Washington and across the USA. Another service is the Speaker's Bureau. This is a free advisory service offered by Berks Cable TV to address issues such as programming, cable TV issues and communications technologies.

Review

Latterly in America, there has been a re-emergence of belief in the need for a (managed) greater public good to operate; one in which more can be winners, and less can be losers. For greater public good to occur, markets have to managed so that all partners can benefit. Realizing this principle, the mayor traded with a commercial company to get maximum advantage for citizens. This, in part, accounts for the success of BCTV.

Long-term success, however, requires more than just 'doing the deal'. Responsive, accessible and equitable ways of sustaining social innovations need to evolve. The BCTV case study demonstrates this convincingly.

Summary

Impressions gained on the visits made to both Facing the Future and Berks Community TV were that the success of both innovations can be traced back to:

- an extremely strong sense of entrepreneurial spirit
- a shared vision about the direction and value of the project
- openness and flexibility in organizational management
- a commitment to bringing free speech and active participation in decision making to the community.

The North American population is at home with technology. All sections of the community, from teenagers through to 'seniors', take its use as a matter of course. Being comfortable with it, they are more likely to use it in innovative ways. The very low costs are also an incentive, whereas in Europe, telephone costs in particular are prohibitive to the full participation of some sectors of the community.

Government works with industry in North America to ensure that, if cable TV licences are granted, the company puts something of value into the community as an exchange. This is a practice that European policy makers should seek to emulate.

9 Promoting Good Practice in Telehealth

'Health is created and lived by people within the settings of their everyday life, where they live, work, play and love. Health is created by caring for oneself and others, by being able to take decisions and have control over one's life circumstances, and by ensuring that the society one lives in creates conditions that allow the attainment of health by all its members.'

(Ottawa Charter, 1986)

Technological advances in medical care and sophisticated hospital care have contributed to a dramatic rise in expenditure on health care in Europe, yet increased spending on health care, technological developments and greater research have not improved the health of the European people as much as might have been expected. There is now increasing recognition (Dutton, 1988; Konner, 1993) that, as far as medical potential in this century is concerned, the wrong choice was made. Instead of investing most of the money and most of the effort in 'after the event' illness care, it should have been invested in 'before the event' preventive care. If it had been, the health profile in European countries today would look markedly different.

In choosing (almost exclusively) to align itself with the 'hard' sciences, medicine in the twentieth century has given greater precedence to the body and its functioning than to the person and his or her well-being. To a very large extent, the reason for this has been the rapid growth and adoption of medical technology, particularly of the 'gee whiz' type (high technology and glamorous at first sight, but often with very limited application and effectiveness in a larger perspective). 'Gee whiz' type technology makes the news, and influences public consciousness and expectations. This, combined with the fact that prevention has been a low status activity, has led people to believe in both the invincibility of medicine, and of life itself. Konner comments:

'Doctors and patients alike wait until illness has reached an advanced stage and then look for a quick fix, one that can often cost a fortune and still not work. Almost all of us overestimate what modern medicine can do, and few of us are prepared to face a fact that people in past generations simply could not ignore: all of us must die sometime.'

In addition to length of life, quality is also important. Milio (1986) commented:

> 'In one sense the medical model is well suited to digitalized information processing . . . but an acknowledged problem in expert system programming is how to integrate contextual data on the breadth of people's lives in order to make sense of effective symptoms and to arrive at a solution. The narrow and rigid filter of the medical model (in a telematics application) is increasingly recognized as inadequate.'

In the same paper, Milio goes on to argue the case for a broader vision, and for health promotion type solutions.

Information technology potential in health care

Nancy Milio is one of few researchers working in the field of telehealth at this time. She has profound and well developed views on the potential offered by information technology (IT) in health care. She was therefore interviewed in March 1993. These are some of her comments:

> 'IT is a set of tools that can be used, if it's used properly . . . in the US, and in Europe also, IT has been used almost entirely, really, for the big players through federal research and grants and software that is useful for hospital systems, and mainly for administrative purposes, just doing the same thing, electronically, that you used to have a horde of clerks doing.
>
> It's very easy for computer technicians to take catalogues and copy them, but to do what you (the author) are talking about means you have to go out and get at the concept of what it's like to be disabled, and ask: what are your problems and what information do you need? And then you have to get somebody to gather that information and put it together in some fashion that makes it highly friendly to the people who will use it. That is a whole other way of thinking, and computer and other experts are often digital thinkers.
>
> What we're talking about is analogue, right brain thinking. It's much more time consuming. It's people oriented. You don't have problems with people if you just turn on these beautiful computer screens, they're wonderful really, but you might as well just have a quick library search, which does serve its purposes. That's doing what we've always done, but doing it electronically.
>
> The point of the new technology is that we can do many more things . . . that we cannot (now) even imagine. The problem is too, that no-one is getting in there with the creative ideas, or nobody that counts!'

The 'nobodies' referred to above are the users. It is time they were placed up front, so this chapter focuses on them.

In previous chapters, users have been separated out in terms of the services they were receiving. Here it is logical to continue to discuss groups of users in terms of the types of need they represent. In doing so, however the object is not to indicate that certain categories of user require (exclusively) certain kinds of provision; in fact the reverse is true. As will be identified later, services developed for one group of people could very well benefit others. Categories of use therefore should be seen as simply a convenient way of presenting information pertaining to the main group of users for whom the service was developed.

Services for women with high risk pregnancies

Case study data suggest that domiciliary fetal monitoring (DFM), as part of an integrated domiciliary antenatal care scheme, is a model of good practice that can and should be extended to other antenatal care service organizations. This finding is in line with that of Hill *et al.* (1990). It is effective, reflects a high degree of user responsiveness, is relatively cheap and easy to use, and is well accepted in practice by service providers and by users. The model of health on which care is based is social rather than exclusively medical, and the reorientation to PHC called for in the Ottawa Charter is evident.

An evaluation of both the economic and social costs of the scheme in Wales is currently occurring, but the data obtained from this case study imply that DFM could be a more cost-efficient form of antenatal care for high risk pregnant women than hospitalization, with its attendant in-patient costs. In addition to costs incurred by the health service, it is also necessary to take into account costs borne by families. There is no doubt that DFM is a lower cost solution for them than in-patient care.

Whilst hard evidence about costs in both urban and rural areas is not yet available, all participants referred to the particular value of DFM in remote rural areas, where public transport is either poor or non-existent. Lack of transport has a 'knock on' effect for families when women are required to have frequent out-patient appointments or be hospitalized (eg childcare, subsistence and visiting costs). Following a recent review of midwifery services in the UK, the Select Committee (Winterton) report (HMSO, 1992) noted that:

'Antenatal visits often involve long and expensive journeys, sometimes with young children in tow. This evidence is borne out in surveys undertaken by Community Health Councils; travelling costs, time and childcare facilities all need to be borne in mind by the service providers at the planning stage if women are not to be discouraged from attending.'

In the same report, recommendations were made on patient ownership of records and continuity of care:

'We conclude that many women at present feel that they are denied access to information in the antenatal period which would enable them to make truly informed choices about their care, their carer and the place of birth. They are unnecessarily deprived of access to their medical notes. Too often bad news is given in an unsympathetic way. Too often they experience an unwillingness on the part of professionals to treat them as equal partners in making decisions . . . Continuity of care in these circumstances is likely to be facilitated by encouraging women to hold their own notes.'

Continuity of care requires teamworking. For teamwork to be effective, there needs to be a shared vision of care and the development, and use, of a care management protocol which recognizes and utilizes resources effectively. Indications are that some obstetricians and midwives will need to work more closely together to maximize the potential offered by DFM. This will necessitate attitude shifs in relation to:

• a more selective use of DFM

• development of integrated care teams.

Referring to provision of the DFM scheme and the need for teamwork, a senior official of the Royal College of Midwives (RCM) said:

'I think it's an excellent idea, it gives more control to mothers. It's not been picked up a lot. It don't know why because it's not expensive . . . the idea seems a great one . . . it prevents women having to trail into hospital just for monitoring. I have no difficulty in supporting the idea. I don't see the need for EFM (electro-fetal monitoring) for all women, only high risk women. It *does* devolve power away from the consultant unit. They are powerful gatekeepers. The politics (surrounding DFM) might reflect the low status of a female profession and doctors fearing the loss of control of care.'

Midwifery services in Europe

Organization of antenatal care differs between European countries. In those countries where midwifery services are provided, they are highly valued by users. Generally, midwifery services are more developed in the northern European countries. It could be argued that it doesn't matter who provides the service as long as it is provided, but in countries where obstetricians dominate service provision, service seems to be medically rather than socially oriented. Whilst no hard data on cost comparisons exist, it is likely that medically oriented services are more expensive. They may also lack service continuity.

In Germany, for example, there are many gynaecologists in private practice; most women attend a gynaecology practice for their antenatal care and then go to hospital for delivery. There are reported to be no means of communication between the gynaecologist and the hospital apart from the co-operation card. This leads to a lack of continuity of care. Since most women do not come across a midwife during pregnancy, they receive very little health promotion advice (Toussaint, 1991).

Organization of maternity care in The Netherlands is reported as being more community oriented; for example, one third of all births occur at home. Sensitive and sensible use of support technologies can support this trend. Births at home save on expensive hospital care, are consumer oriented and offer pregnant women more freedom of choice (Teijlingen, 1989).

There is a move towards community based practice in Denmark, particularly in rural areas. Here midwives work in 'midwifery centres' situated in the community. They offer antenatal care and parentcraft classes. Clausen (1992) reports that it is usual for a midwife to work one day a week in the centre, and the rest of the week on the labour ward of the local hospital.

Spain has recently recommenced midwifery training and, especially in rural areas, is moving towards an integrated system of care with the development of primary health care teams.

French midwifery is said to be limited by obstetric practices (Tagawa, 1992). Greece, Portugal, and Italy too, as is the case in Germany, are reported as having services based on the medical model of care.

It appears that those countries that provide antenatal care by means of midwifery rather than obstetric services offer a service that is more socially oriented, appropriate and acceptable to women themselves. It is therefore recommended that midwifery services should be offered in all EU countries as part of integrated antenatal care provision, and should be clearly based on agreed protocols of antenatal care management. These should include effective and efficient use of appropriate support technologies.

Telephones as medical equipment

For some pregnant women, the most vital piece of support technology is the telephone. Ironically those most in need of telephone services (economically disadvantaged 'high risk' pregnant women) were found to be least likely to own them. In this instance, for preventive surveillance, a telephone should be regarded as a medical appliance, and treated as such. Telephones should be purchased by health authorities and made available for loan for the duration of need, the way any other piece of medical equipment is loaned (eg a wheelchair or walking frame). As both high risk pregnancies and non-telephone ownership affect only a very small number of the total population of pregnant women, the cost will be low, and certainly cheaper than the cost of hospitalization. Mobile telephones would be ideal for the purpose as neither installation nor disconnection costs would be incurred.

Services for adolescents

The decision to study health promotion with adolescents was prompted by the health potential they represent. They present our greatest opportunity for achieving a healthier future. These young people are the parents, citizens and leaders of tomorrow (UNICEF/WHO, 1992).

If the goal is to promote the health of young citizens, two things need to be recognized:

1 Health promotion interventions need to relate to the lifestyles of young people.

2 They need to be offered in a format which is preferred by young people.

Both criteria are met by the E ZOOT initiative in Canada. A range of 'youth friendly' formats is offered, centred on provision of both a youth magazine and an electronic Bulletin Board. These initiatives are supported by an extensive network of community development activities, all aimed to promote adolescent health and reduce adolescent threats to health.

Major risks for young people are substance abuse (alcohol, tobacco, 'soft' and 'hard' drugs) and sexually transmitted diseases including AIDS. Young people with low self-esteem are more likely to take health risks than those with high self-esteem. Moreover, youngsters who take one health risk are more likely to take others (ie are susceptible to a cluster of threats). The behaviour change approach that offers most chance of success with these young people is a broad based 'lifeskills' approach which builds self-esteem and thus equips youngsters to cope with a range of threatening situations, rather than just one.

'Lifeskills' for behaviour change

At E ZOOT, a lifeskills approach is employed to promote the building of mature, reflective behaviour. The indications are that this socially responsive health promotion approach is more likely to reduce sustained behaviour change than the narrow, medically based, negative risk reduction approaches that are the norm in so many European health education campaigns.

Hansen *et al.* (1991) report findings from a project similar to the E ZOOT one, which had the goal of reducing drug use:

'The findings of this study suggest that the key to changing substance abuse patterns (legal and illegal drugs) requires changing sociological factors that account for the onset of use . . . in particular, establishing conservative norms within adolescent friendship groups may effectively reduce demands that otherwise may serve to promote substance use.'

Nutbeam *et al.* (1991) have commented that traditional health education campaigns appear very naive in their approach to influencing health behaviour among young people. They are seen as naive in terms of both the message and the form of provision (ie mass media, 'top down', individualistic, education programmes). According to Castanheira (1991):

'Most of the programmes to promote adolescent health are neither on the right track nor going in the right direction. The right track for health promotion is the community.'

At E ZOOT a social model of health is used and exploited to its full potential. Additionally, service provision has been reoriented towards community responsive health promotion. The creation of supportive environments for the making of healthy lifestyle choices is also evident, as is collaboration with other providers and networks to develop healthy public policy.

Service costs are very low; vision, direction and commitment are very high. The service began modestly and planned growth is also modest and in line with the quality of service staff know they can deliver within budget limitations. It is gratifying to note that, although the sponsoring agency (AADAC) has suffered a budget cut, E ZOOT work has been protected.

It is impressive to reflect on what the E ZOOT team have achieved with limited resources. Their success must be seen as largely due to the existence of an open management style, in which risks are taken, creativity is supported and everyone's contribution is valued. A large part of E ZOOT's success is due to teamwork. The team not only models good intra-team skills, but also good extra-team (networking) skills in the way it works with other organizations (eg schools, parents and police) to build a shared vision of the health potential of young Albertans.

Services for disabled people

The Europe wide information system for the disabled (HANDYNET) forms a direct contrast to E ZOOT. It is larger, vastly more expensive and (as it currently stands) less effective. Perhaps the most striking thing about HANDYNET is the lack of involvement of users in the system. Whilst a real information need exists, which could be addressed, HANDYNET and user organizations operate in isolation to each other. Exactly who HANDYNET is meant to serve remains unclear. The HELIOS literature certainly sees it as a resource for users as well as professionals. However, Humphreys (1992) says:

> 'Few of HANDYNET's 30 million intended beneficiaries are aware of its existence . . . if it is to benefit people with disabilities all over Europe, as it intends, it needs to make real use of its human assets. It needs to concentrate less on rhetoric and more on reality.'

The evidence indicated by the data collected for this project is that, where users are aware of HANDYNET's existence, they perceive it as a resource for professionals. They also see it as being largely irrelevant to their need. As it is currently constructed, HANDYNET seems to be a scheme constructed by providers for providers. This is particularly regrettable in view of the 'good practice' in service provision that was found to exist in the host institutions visited in Italy and The Netherlands. A disabilities researcher concluded:

> 'My feeling is that the HANDYNET project is too big, ambitious and complicated, and suffered in the early stages from being technology driven rather than an idea of what was useful, or indeed possible . . . the differences in funding source may be a contributory factor too . . . Since national funding depends on individual governments, there are considerable differences between countries in the extent of support available, as well as between the national centres and Brussels. To someone accustomed to "shoestring" activities in the voluntary sector, the Brussels approach can seem quite extravagant.'

For their effective use, information systems need to offer, in addition to availability and accessibility, information that is worth accessing.

Information so far collected for HANDYNET is in the subject area 'equipment for people with disabilities'. Perhaps this was the easiest place to start, but this type of application only uses a fraction of the potential available to the format. The operating system (CD-ROM) is capable technologically, of much more than its current application, generating masses of catalogue type product data. The main advantage is that what might take up a wall of shelves in a library is contained on a tiny lightweight disc. However, whilst the type of information being offered is important, it addresses only a narrow area of need. A person may buy, at most, three wheelchairs in his life; on the other hand, he or she may have 10 jobs and numerous sport and leisure opportunities. Realization of this fact may be behind the view expressed in a COST 219 publication, that:

> 'work with HANDYNET has been going on for several years without showing much progress'. (Tetzchner, 1991)

However, as one interviewee pointed out, development work takes time, and so does building international co-operation. It also helps to have a secure operating framework, in this case HELIOS. It must be said that, since HELIOS began managing HANDYNET, there is both greater international effectiveness and awareness of the need to involve users. The Commission's recent decision in 1993, to limit current development work to the Technical Aids module, is therefore highly regrettable.

It has not been possible to get full details of costs, but the duration (it began in 1986) and scale of HANDYNET work indicate that fairly substantial costs will have been involved. A better decision, with regard to effectiveness as well as efficiency, might have been to fund more collaborative pilot work in fewer countries, on two modules. In addition to Technical Aids, for example, another module (with user involvement) could have explored pan European social data, such as employment or leisure opportunities and legislation.

The current format (on its own) and the choice of module have not encouraged social integration. In addition to developing further models relating to the social (as opposed to the medical aspects) of everyday life, other formats (such as the E Mail facility) should be explored so that users can themselves enter and 'own' data, for example on product evaluations and travel tips. In these circumstances a live accessible format, such as an electronic bulletin board, would be more appropriate than CD-ROM. Such developments could be embraced in the latest HANDYNET related Commission recommendations (1993), which advocate:

> 'positive and forward looking activities to encourage the adaption of technologies, including new technologies, to the needs of disabled people'.

Elderly people: social support for independent living

In the EU, the elderly population will total 56 million by the year 2000, and the disabled will total 36–48 million (OECD, 1988) Owing to the changing demographic structure of Europe, support of the elderly and those with special needs is now a major policy issue for health care providers. In particular, the need for social services is growing. Currently this need is realized through regular domiciliary visits, 'sheltered' housing schemes and residential (institutional) care. All the evidence to date (Ballabio *et al.*, 1992) suggests that this latter option is the one least preferred by users. Case study visits to The Netherlands, Germany, Portugal and Canada support this assertion.

Two case studies explored support systems to promote independent living: personal alarms and videotelephony. Whilst both are used principally to support elderly people living at home, they have the potential to provide either permanent or temporary support to all citizens in need.

Alarm systems

The current policy trend in Europe is to promote care in the community, rather than in institutions. Provision of remote alarm services for citizens in need supports this policy. Services offer most potential, and may be most cost-effective, when offered as part of an integrated care package. Fragmentation of service delivery systems and financing arrangements threatens the goal of integrated care. Increased fragmentation of services is likely with the introduction of market principles into health care.

As with other preventive primary health promotion schemes, costs to government are difficult to establish. However, as with the domiciliary fetal monitoring scheme, it can be assumed that out-patient community support costs will be less than in-patient care or full institutional support (ie nursing home) costs.

Alarm systems are a relatively cheap and effective aid to support independent living. They have two main benefits for users: firstly, they give a feeling of safety to individuals; secondly, they make organization of adequate help possible in the (usually rare) times of emergency. They can support independent living in all types of individuals and families, from premature babies through to the frail elderly. They may also have a role to play in early discharge of patients back into the community following (ever briefer) periods of hospitalization. Use of medical technology means that more infants become viable and more people can live longer. Alarm systems offer user friendly low technology support for independent living in the community.

Videotelephony

Some citizens need more in terms of social support than alarm systems can offer. Videotelephony (VT) services may be a more cost-effective form of care provision than either institutional care or provision of domiciliary visiting services. In addition, a well planned and delivered VT service increases the potential for teamwork. Better use can be made of the professional skills of different care team members, and service provision can be maximized. Services (such as gymnastics or religious worship) that are offered in the care settings that double as VT service centres can be transmitted (live or on videotape) to the broader user audience in the community. This makes the service both more equitable and more cost-effective.

Evaluation of the service pilots (RACE project 1054, 1993) reports that users like the service and want more of it. Service providers were also satisfied:

> 'They are optimistic about the practical viability of service provision via videotelephony . . . They feel that visual contact is more satisfactory and more informative. Videotelephony reduces their travel needs and therefore saves time and increases their ability to service clients' true needs.' (evaluator)

It has been alleged (Cullan *et al.*, 1991) that a major potential risk with new technology is the risk of social isolation. However, videotelephony may on the contrary, have the potential to increase, rather than diminish, social presence. Data collected show that videotelephony has the potential to extend social networks for the housebound. It also has the potential to form an electronic substitute for face-to-face visiting and provision of remote care services.

Provision of both remote alarm services and videotelephony services support independent living in the community. Their potential is exciting. They should be viewed as proactive rather than reactive services, for groups of citizens who may otherwise not be very visible in public life (the 'shut-ins'). Policy makers and health professionals need to promote the active participation of these citizens in community life by integrating electronic service provision with face-to-face service provision where appropriate, and with involvement in social events (eg bussing service users to special events, such as senior citizens' Christmas parties).

Telehealth, citizens and public policy making

This chapter began by commenting on the route taken by medicine in the twentieth century. Social policy, by default, has allowed disproportionate accretion of power to the medical profession. There is now a real danger of investing in technologists the same type of hegemonic power that has been invested in doctors for most of this century. The way to avoid that is to invest in and revalue citizens, and offer them opportunities to take a full and active part in decision making.

Before they can participate, citizens need information. Gann (1991) comments that information may not automatically lead to health, but without information consumers cannot take the first step. Roling (1992) also sees involvement of citizens as necessary:

> '. . . authorities and professionals do not "own" health. In fact, old procedures and scientific insights can prove seriously out of date and no longer suitable for dealing with modern hazards. We live in an era of discontinuity, and science and established procedure can no longer be relied upon to provide all the answers . . . citizens are active in creating meaning for the events around them. It is useful to look on them as activists . . . such an attitude towards citizens seems more fruitful than looking at them as clients, patients or customers.'

Milio (1992) quotes community action literature which suggests that collective use of new technologies can both build and bind communities. Reviewing a number of studies in the USA, she says:

> 'Information technology has been the impetus for collective action, including establishing collective ties between local groups and policy makers, influencing public opinion, and bringing improvements in local resources and policy implementation.'

The North American population is at home with technology. All sections of the community, from teenagers through to 'seniors', take its use as a matter of course. Being comfortable with it, they are more likely to use it in innovative ways. The very low costs are also an incentive, whereas in Europe, telephone costs in particular are prohibitive to the full participation of some sectors of the community.

Government works with industry in North America to ensure that, if licences are granted (eg for cable TV), the company puts something of value into the community as an exchange. This is a practice European policy makers should seek to emulate. In The Netherlands they are already moving in this direction:

> 'In close dialogue with the central office of the Unions of the Elderly, and in dialogue with other organizations of the elderly, approaches will be sought to increase their opportunities to make their own choices. This should probably be done through this group's own leaders of opinion, older persons who can show how they have dealt with choice problems in their own situations. Perhaps something can be done using an interactive approach through afternoon television.' (Ministry of Health, 1992)

The videotelephony and the 'teledemocracy' case studies indicate that this approach could be successful. Success, however, should not be measured in audience participation figures (the traditional way of measuring broadcasting success), but by one of a number of social indicators designed to measure the health and well-being of a population subgroup.

The technologies

The focus of this book is sociological rather than technical. Those who wish to understand more fully details of technological innovations are referred to Veneris (1992). Technologists have been particularly helpful, however, in identifying the possibilities and limitations of certain technologies. In addition to assistance during case study visits, they have helped clarify issues during the final drafting stages of this book.

Integrated services digital networks (ISDN)

In their view, the most significant current telecommunications innovation is the advent of integrated services digital networks (ISDN). Giles and Lewis (1992) explain why:

> 'The network is digital and has been for some time. The local loop . . . the bit of wire which runs from the exchange to a customer . . . has always been analogue. Irrespective of the equipment linked to the phone line . . . the message leaves the premises as an analogue signal . . . it travels to the exchange at the edge of the network, which digitizes it. It then travels across the network as a digital signal until it reaches the exchange on the other side of the network. The receiving exchange converts it back to analogue to travel the final distance along the local loop to the called party. If the analogue local loop carried digital signals, instead of conversion at the exchange and then back again at the other end, the signal could run digitally from end to end. The Industry designed ISDN to do just that.'

So ISDN is a 'smart' system that facilitates a wide range of technological uses. Provision of ISDN facilities is related to the state of provision of telephone services. Telephone communications are said to be more widely available and more advanced in northern Europe than in the south. European standards for ISDN are in place and availability in the North will shortly be 100%. Availability in major centres in the South will also soon be achieved (information given by a member of the EC Telematics Working Group, June 1993).

CD-ROM

With one exception, all of the technological innovations explored in this book will rely on ISDN development. The exception is CD-ROM, the main medium selected by HANDYNET. A European technical expert was asked (June 1993) about the relationship between CD-ROM and ISDN. He replied:

'That's not easy to answer, or to see. There *is* a use but it's a "bolt on" supplementary, rather than an integral part of the system.'

He went on to discuss possible limitations of CD-ROM, as far as users are concerned:

'CD-ROM is good for huge databases and directories. A problem with CD-ROM is that you only get what's put in, and that relies on who puts it in. Consumers cannot send queries and information back. Its best use is for huge amounts of data that change very little . . . but if you need to update you can send out E Mail, or post a floppy (disc).'

If the need is purely for information (as opposed to interaction), CD-ROM holds vast technical potential:

'One CD-ROM can hold more than 600 megabytes of text, graphics, music, maps, moving video, computer programs and other digital data, so there's almost no limit to what can be served up on a silver platter. And since it costs less than £1 (UK) to press a CD, huge quantities of material could be distributed at a very low price.' (Schofield, 1993)

Guidance for decision making

It is further reported, however, that hardware and software incompatibilities stand between this dream and the reality, and that further manufacturers' technology wars loom. During this time it will be very difficult for policy makers to make decisions about use of appropriate technology. Nevertheless Dutton (1988) offers guidance. Based on her case study analysis of four technological innovations, she has identified the common pitfalls in decision making as:

- technological optimism (in which potential benefits are stressed and potential problems minimalized)

- underestimation of risk (in which no evidence of risk is taken as evidence of no risk)

- suppression of doubt and dissent (in which uncertainties and controversies are suppressed)

- 'hard' data dwarfing 'soft' concerns (in which technical aspects are accorded more status than social, ethical and political ones)

- a fragmentary and myopic view of problems (in which the complexity of biomedical issues encourages reductionist thinking)

- assumption of unlimited resources (in which piecemeal budgetary decisions are made without recourse to policy priorities)

- inflexibility of decisions (in which the originators of innovations resist changes and 'interference').

Policy makers and service planners should bear these pitfalls in mind when commissioning research and service provision.

With regard to research into the health potential offered by new technologies, almost all the funding for 'health' research is allocated to the medical technologies. The effect of this is to promote glamorous high technology innovations as scientific breakthroughs (Gelijne and Halm, 1991). The research funding balance needs to be redressed in favour of telehealth as opposed to telemedicine, and the role of social technologies more fully explored.

In terms of commissioning, reductionist thinking can lead to opportunities being lost. At a recent technology conference (InterCHI, 1993), Newell attacked technologists' obsession with the 'average' user and pointed out that creativity needs to be encouraged and novel applications recognized. He cited hearing aids as the first major market for micro-electronics, the cassette tape recorder as a solution for blind people, and the TV remote control device as a solution for the mobility impaired. All originated from small user sensitive projects and all now have huge market shares.

Summary

During the twentieth century, medicine has served the interests of professionals rather than citizens. There is a danger that, unchecked, health care in the twenty-first century will become dominated by a different type of professional, the technocrat. The dangers inherent in this are that:

1 technologists may miss the mark altogether, as far as societies' needs are concerned

2 they may focus exclusively on innovations with narrow applications.

Technologists need to begin their work by consulting users and continue to work with them to come up with relevant solutions to meet their needs. E ZOOT started off with a user problem and looked for an appropriate solution; it is very successful. HANDYNET started off with an application and looked for a problem to apply it to; it has subsequently been much less successful.

Striking characteristics of successful case studies have been:

- use of a Health For All orientation
- the ability to work with, rather than at people
- appropriate use of technology.

10 Telehealth For All

'. . . the point of the new technologies is that we can do many more things . . .'

(Milio, interview data, 1993)

Telehealth involves the promotion and facilitation of health and well-being with individuals and communities, by use of telematic services. The case studies explored in this book demonstrate the potential that telehealth has to promote health and well-being, and offer ideas for new and exciting ways forward in telematics for health.

In analysing good practice in telehealth, an exploration of the philosophical rationales on which various practices have been based was necessary. Unequivocally, best practice is based on Health For All principles.

Health choices

Health For All is a worldwide movement aimed at reorienting health services towards primary health care and prevention of ill health, as opposed to the promise of cure. As disenchantment with the 'magic bullet' approach to health, sets in, governments worldwide are seeking a different base for health care policy making. Europe, in this context, is leading the way and providing role models. From the health care reforms in the USA (National Issues Forum Institute, 1992; OTA, 1991; National Information Infrastructure, 1993) to the development of a national primary health care policy in Australia (CDHH&S, 1993; Sax, 1990), Health For All values, originating in the European office of the World Health Organization, are being adopted.

Increasingly, it is recognized that there are many causal factors in health, and the provision of medical care is only one of them. This recognition has sparked off a very welcome international debate about health choices. It has to be recognized, however, that the origins of the debate have not been entirely altruistic. What has grabbed the attention of policy makers has been the rapidly escalating cost of medical technology, which, if unchecked, threatens to destabilize and even consume entire health budgets. Concomitant with the rise in the cost of medical technologies has been a rise in the expectations of the general public. Quality of life is a major casualty of these raised expectations.

Unrealistic expectations

Burnett (1978) has suggested that the predominant attitude of society at present is that every individual is entitled to go on living, at whatever cost to families and communities, and that the primary purpose of medical care is to let this be achieved. There are occasions, he alleges, when purpose 'excessive investigation and treatment, including discomfort, indignity and pain, do little more than fill the interval to death'.

How did we arrive at the above scenario? An answer to this question can be found by identifying the often hidden incentives in health care systems that encourage inappropriate budgeting and technological choices. These include technological optimism, underestimation of risk and suppression of dissent used to 'sell' medical technology, as identified by Dutton (*see*

pages 132, 133), and the prevailing 'gee whiz' medical and public appreciation of technology cited by the Visiting Fogarty Fellow (DFM case study, *see*
page 42) during data collection for this study:

> '. . . then there's the "gee whizz factor" . . . we've got this incredible
> thing . . . gee whiz: let's have one on the health service.'

Prevention with primary health care

It is a truism, well known to primary health care workers, that prevention is
not glamorous. Therefore, it has not been attention grabbing as far as either
the general public or health care policy makers are concerned. However,
there is now a different mood amongst health care policy makers, and
prevention is now centre stage, although a cautionary approach prevails and
change is largely still at the rhetorical stage. This is because of a general
reluctance to fund primary health care (PHC) adequately.

Reorienting health services towards PHC means putting more money into
PHC and less into hospital high technology care. Prevention is more useful
than state of the art and sometimes spurious diagnostic and monitoring
activities. Ironically, high technology care is not subjected to the same
scrutiny, with regard to effectiveness and efficiency, that PHC generally is. In
the few instances that the cost and efficiency of PHC (as opposed to hospital
care) has been explored, PHC has been found to be superior:

> 'Particularly in respect of life expectancy, Norway's historical bias towards
> primary care has produced similar results to those of Sweden, where
> hospital treatment has traditionally been more prominent. The per capita
> cost of health care, however, has been significantly lower in Norway than
> in Sweden. The differences in policy between the two countries largely
> explains the lower per capita cost of Norway's health system. Given the
> approximately equal mortality rates, it seems that the Norwegian system,
> with its emphasis on primary care, is the more effective.' (Agdestein and
> Roemer, 1991)

Others (Greenland, 1990; Callaghan, 1993) also argue the case for investing
in PHC. However, Rosen and Lindholm (1992) caution that direct comparison
of PHC investment and outcome is not a simple equation:

> 'A review of cost-effectiveness and cost utility analysis studies applied to
> health promotion, and lifestyle interventions in particular, indicates that
> many benefits and some risks of these measures are not considered in the
> analyses. This may bias the results and lead to less than optimal use of
> available resources. The basic measure of health benefits has usually been

mortality for a single disease, in spite of the fact that a change in lifestyle may well change the incidence of morbidity for other diseases as well. Beneficial effects on the incidence and duration of non-fatal diseases are often disregarded.'

Rosen and Lindholm, additionally indicate that we should broaden our gaze in terms of understanding cause and effect relationships and the methods used to collect data. Green (1991) also sees current medical research methodologies as having limited potential, and argues for a phenomenological approach:

'The problem with measurement and controlled experimental or statistical testing of theories as criteria of their relative worth, is that these criteria bias the selection toward the more simplistic or mechanistic slices of reality. Reductionism becomes rampant; empiricism becomes imperial; technology becomes technocracy. One's most powerful research tools are one's eyes and ears, wired to one's thinking apparatus.'

A plea for eclecticism in the use of indicators has also been made by Henderson (1993), when talking about the need to redefine wealth and progress and thus build back quality in society:

'Why not let's just have unbundled indicators; dozens and dozens of them if necessary, which show us all kinds of aspects and quality of life and help us to deal with these quality of life dimensions directly . . . and build our coalitions around them, and in this way, if you're interested in education you can watch literacy rates and how many children are in headstart programmes, and if you care about the environment you can watch the air quality index from the top of a building in a city like Sao Paolo or New York, and if you're concerned with species loss you can watch the indicators of how fast that is going. In other words we really don't need economists anymore . . . to go in the back room and to do all of this weighting using their arcane formulae and coming up with this aggregation of all these apples and oranges into one single indicator.' (transcript of plenary)

Policies for health

It is evident from the above that, as health choices must continue to be made, some of the criteria on which they are currently based deserve closer scrutiny. Service costs and associated outcomes are very difficult to quantify, but with soaring expenditure on health (illness) care in all EU countries, cost-effectiveness and efficiency need to be addressed.

The current trend seems to be the introduction of market principles into provision of health services. Either these can be allowed to operate freely (as they have, disastrously, in the USA), or they can be managed, as they have been in the British National Health Service (NHS). Ironically, just as the USA is taking on the massive challenge of its health service reforms with the goal of making them more like the NHS, Britain, together with other European countries, is introducing more competition into health care, thus fragmenting it. The problem with government attempts to bring the commercial ethic into public services is that governments have to provide services which no sane commercial organization would undertake. In public sector provision, moral and social imperatives need to be combined with economic ones.

Public/private and inter-agency collaboration

In planning future health services, European policy makers need to stimulate the public and the private sector to work more closely together. They also need to be aware that health services need not exclusively be defined as medical services; as we have seen in the case studies, social technologies can promote health efficiently and effectively. They may also have a better health 'pay off' than medical technologies.

A broad vision and effective inter-agency collaboration are needed if governments are to realize fully their collaborative potential with private enterprise. The French Government, with its integrated public/private approach to building low cost, safe 'smart' homes is showing the way. By installing additional telephone cables into 7000 domestic flats at Chateauroux, the French Government is providing security and support for independent living for its citizens. Alarms, bulletin boards (Minitel) and videophone services are included; the cost is said to be around £500 (650 ECU) per flat (Computer Guardian, 10.3.94).

Vision and entrepreneurial skills are also necessary to prevent the 'turf wars' of unchecked private enterprise occurring, together with the massive financial losses that ensue, with concomitant dissipation of energy, skills and goodwill. Europe would do well to look to North America if it is to improve its entrepreneurial skills. Although a competitive market economy characterizes North American society, competition doesn't necessarily mean only a few have to win. There is a feature of North American society that is worth emulating: its ability to produce situations where all the participants benefit. Case study data (E ZOOT, Reading citizen's TV) demonstrate the validity of the entrepreneurial approach. It was also advocated by the Visiting Fogarty Fellow to the UK, who, whilst extolling the virtues of the British PHC system, remarked:

'I didn't expect each unit to be doing its own thing. You do wonder why, if you have a system like this (DFM), where you potentially could have some centralization, there are not some recommendations from central Government saying, these are the ones that we approve, recommend, and authorize, and we've worked out a special deal with the manufacturers to get you a price break.'

Collaboration and co-ordination of the type that is being advocated is now evident in the EU *Fourth framework programme for community research and technological development (1994–98)*. This recognizes that telematics can be used to offer various categories of users, particularly public services and private individuals, new ranges of products and services to meet basic economic and social requirements:

'Research in the field of telematic applications in areas of common interest will have two aims. One will be to promote the competitiveness of European industry . . . the other . . . is to promote research activities necessary for other common policies . . . more importance will be attached to user requirements and the search for the most efficient and economical solutions possible.' (CEC [1993] 459)

The programme, as proposed, should help promote sensible and sensitive use of telematics for the promotion of health and well-being, and reduce the incidence of HANDYNET type scenarios in the future.

The *Framework for action in the field of public health* (CEC [1993] 559) sets out the Commission's proposals for taking forward the Community's work on public health to meet the objective introduced by the Treaty on European Union that 'the Community shall contribute towards ensuring a high level of human health protection'. The approach will include the establishment of common objectives and networks, exchange of information and personnel, improvement of data systems, financial support to programmes and projects, production of an annual Community health report, and assistance to cost reduction efforts.

One project where collaboration between EU divisions and project teams is already evident is the European Prototype for Integrated Care (EPIC) project. The aim of EPIC is to develop a prototype IT infrastructure capable of supporting the delivery of health and social care to enable people to maintain optimal quality of their lives in their own home environments. While this project will concentrate on care of the elderly, it is the intention that it could be applicable, with minimal adjustment, to other vulnerable client groups in the future (Boydell, 1992).

People consultation

In addition to greater collaboration and better resource use between funders and service providers, there needs to be recognition and use of the resources that 'ordinary people' possess. This resource base is vast and remains un-tapped, largely because of prejudice and paternalism. The demographic increase in the number of elderly people that Europe is currently experiencing is a good case in point. Young and Schuller (1991) argue:

> 'Old age could once be regarded as a sort of terminal illness; it cannot any longer. The globe has been pulled together into one network by specialized communications, but pulled apart by new and equally specialized institu-tions for industry and education, health and amusement, which have taken over what the family, as an all-age affair, once did largely on its own . . . when the clock strikes 65 (years), the magic wand of the State turns not coachmen into mice but men (workers) into old men . . . age stratification resembles a caste society in which people are born into a caste, peasants, merchants, nobility . . . the low caste in this instance (are) the young, old, disabled.' (or, in Milio's words,' nobody who matters').

Young and Schuller, in their research study, found two categories of retiree: positive activists and negative isolationists. They also reported the existence of 'positive third agers':

> 'Older people (who) are getting what they can of a positive nature from a stage of life that may well last a quarter of a century or more . . . the most striking fact is that the positive people are engaged in activities, which, in a way, resemble what they did before. Many of them are engaged in "work", although not paid work.'

Third agers represent a major health promotion and health care resource, as do other categories of less visible citizen. One thinks in particular of the highly skilled and active disabled people who participated in this project. These resources need to be recognized by policy makers and service planners.

To ignore the resource that people and communities represent is, in addition to being arrogantly paternalistic, uneconomic. Evidence from the case studies demonstrates that much of the innovative and socially responsive work that occurs in health protection and promotion goes on at local community level. The Healthy Cities movement (*see* Ashton, 1992) is testimony to this approach. Visionaries like Henderson (1993), recognize that 'innovation never comes from the centre, always from the margin'.

During the latter part of this century Western society has become fragmented. The 'we' generations of the post-war and 'hippy' decades have become the 'me' generation of the eighties and early nineties. Social policies have encouraged the cult of selfish individualism. Health policy has become victim blaming, by implying that those who suffer illness are feckless because they do not take better care of themselves. The policy direction that Europe is currently taking with regard to adopting market strategies in provision of health services will compound the damage.

There is a different, and a better way. It is signalled by some related paradigm shifts: *Reinventing government* (Osborne and Gaebler, 1993); *The new public health* (Ashton and Seymour, 1988); *Redefining Wealth and Progress* (Henderson, 1993) and *The spirit of community* (Etzioni, 1993). What binds these movements together is a belief in citizens and their abilities. New thinking about the role of governments sees them as entrepreneurial facilitators, rather than custodians of civic life.

Extensive case study research in the USA has led Osborne and Gaebler (1993) to conclude that the entrepreneurial spirit can transform governments from huge and inefficient bureaucracies into entrepreneurial organizations which can better serve the interests of people and communities. They chronicle (by case study examples) the efforts of hundreds of government officials to bring business technologies to public services.

The New Public Health

Milio (1992) has written about the potential of information technology to improve community involvement in health. She believes that potential uses include:

- organizational uses in support of community groups
- economic capacity building
- health service provision
- community action.

Many of the above activities are encapsulated in the New Public Health movement, derived from Health For All principles.

Social commentators have observed that the New Public Health movement is very like the 'old' (Victorian) public health movement, with its emphasis on governmental and citizens' rights and responsibilities. This is true, and necessary. A feature of all the 'new' movements is that they look back as well as forward. The new economics recognizes the value of other types of social currency than cash and the new communitarian movement recognizes the value of social organization to generate the common good (Etzioni, 1993). Looking back urges us to be cautious about 'progress'. Reviewing Western health care this century, the inescapable conclusion is that the major growth area ('after the event' service provision) got in the way of society's real need: health protection and promotion. As, around the world, health provision is being reappraised, appropriate use of telematic services needs to be debated. It is urged that the potential of social technologies receive more attention from health care policy makers and practitioners than they have done in the past. This might prevent telemedicine from consuming a disproportionate amount of attention and resources, and telehealth from being reinvented some time in the twenty-first century.

Summary

In this chapter, the major themes of this book have been drawn together. A case has been made for the adoption of Health For All principles in policy planning and service delivery, and for expansion of primary health care and community health promotion, supported by appropriate technologies. A strong case has also been made for citizen involvement in health related decision making, and health protection and health promotion activities.

11 Concluding Recommendations

Policy making

The European Commission should promote the sharing of experiences of telematics in health promotion and health care between countries and regions, for example by organizing meetings, facilitating exchange visits, providing a clearing house for information and issuing appropriate publications.

Policy makers (funders and governments) need to be aware that the effectiveness/efficiency potential of telehealth is greater than that of telemedicine, and should commission more research studies in the area of telehealth.

Telematic applications of proven value have been found to be:

- domiciliary fetal monitoring (DFM)
- electronic Bulletin Board Systems (BBS) for youth health promotion
- remote alarm systems for citizens in potential need of emergency services
- videotelephony for social and medical support
- teledemocracy for public participation in decision making.

All of the above innovations need ongoing support and wider dissemination. For full dissemination to occur, the potential of each innovation needs to be recognized. Although a service may have been developed for one particular population group, it may be more generally applicable. For example, remote alarm systems are as useful to the parents of premature infants as they are to the elderly and the disabled.

When a technological application is being developed there should be more communication and collaboration between health service policy makers, health professionals, technologists, health researchers and service users at European, national, regional and local level, with regard to:

- policy making

- service planning

- service delivery

- service evaluation.

Additionally, government at all levels needs to:

- promote the user's right and access to health related information

- seek to promote a more positive view of elderly and disabled people by recognizing and utilizing the vast store of skills and abilities that they possess

- involve the citizens affected by a particular innovation (young, old, pregnant women, disabled) in all aspects of policy making and policy evaluation

- promote the active participation of all citizens in community life by both electronic integration and social integration wherever possible (ie remote health care supported by involvement in social events offered by other care and social institutions).

Policy makers need to accept that technology is only a part of the whole care package, not a substitute for it. Telematics works best when there is a combination of remote and face-to-face servicing, and when there is continuity of care staff, enabling therapeutic relationships to be developed and maintained.

Since budgets are limited, technological innovations should be introduced incrementally, on a small scale, and major commitments and investments should not be made by funding bodies or governments until the proven value of the innovation has been established. An area that funders at all levels should be particularly cautious about is 'risk factor' screening and surveillance.

Policy makers should recognize that much of the really innovative and socially responsive work that occurs in service provision goes on at local community level (DFM, PRISMA, E ZOOT). Funding and government agencies should require evidence of local and national responsiveness and collaboration when funding major programmes, and should also make grants available to smaller local organizations so that good practice can grow and be disseminated.

Practice

At international, national, regional and local level, the Health For All philosophy should be used as a basis for service planning, delivery and evaluation. Government at all these levels therefore needs to recognize that:

1 health and welfare workers in general lack health promotion knowledge and skills

2 true teamwork in primary health care is the exception, rather than the norm

3 until **1** and **2** are addressed, telematics will not be able to achieve its full potential in either health promotion or remote care services.

Training programmes need to be organized to address these deficits. Use of telematic services should also be included in the basic and post basic training of health and welfare professionals. Ideally, training programmes should be multidisciplinary and based on 'problem solving' case study exercises. Each of the six case studies explored in this book could be used for teaching purposes.

A shift in budgetary allocation from hospitals to the primary health care sector could facilitate the development and use of telehealth and remote home care services. Such a shift is recommended.

Health and welfare services do not operate in isolation of other forms of social provision. In the public sector, intersectoral collaboration in provision and use of telematic services will increase their effectiveness and efficiency. Governments should work more closely with the private sector to ensure that the needs of society as well as the needs of industry are being met when products are offered on the market. This will, however, require sensitive collaborative decision making at the European level. An urgent need for policy makers to address is the equitable and economic provision of telephone services throughout the EU. In case studies, some users were disadvantaged and could have been barred from care because they did not possess a telephone. In some circumstances, telephones become a necessary piece of medical equipment. They should be recognized as such and provided accordingly.

Using existing low technology innovations, citizens should be encouraged to participate in decision making with regard to service provision and evaluation. The type (but not degree) of participation that is possible will depend to some extent on the stage of technological development that each country is at (eg percentage of telephone ownership), but citizens of all European countries should be able to participate if the intention is there on the part of government.

Research

Good practice in health related telematics needs to be further identified and disseminated. Comprehensive and complementary identification and dissemination strategies need to be agreed and implemented at international, national, regional and local levels.

In order to understand and appropriately address future health needs, a broad vision rather than a narrow focus is necessary. This requires that project teams be multidisciplinary, and that a range of research methods be used to more fully reflect both the complexity of issues and the future potential of this new paradigm area.

Users' views have been largely ignored to date. An international study of users' perceptions and experiences of telematics should be commissioned by the EC.

Finally, as regards funding for further research and service provision, there are two common questions that policy makers and funders need always to have in mind:

1   Technology for what?

2   Technology for whom?

Appendix: Contact Person by Case Study

Domiciliary fetal monitoring (UK)

Dr Andrew Dawson
Consultant Obstetrician and Gynaecologist
Nevill Hall Hospital
Abergavenny
Gwent NP7 7EG
Wales
United Kingdom
Tel: 0873 852091
Fax: 0873 859168

HANDYNET

The Netherlands

Mr Theo Bougie
HANDYNET Project Co-ordinator
Revalidatie Informatie Centrum
Postbus 88
6430 AB Hoensbroek
Zandsbergsweg 111
6432 Hoensbroek
Netherlands
Tel: +31 45 239360/239369

MS Marry van Dongen
Dutch Independent Living Movement
Moermond 27
333CL Zwijndrecht
Netherlands
Tel: +31 78 127333

Italy

Mr Renzo Andrich
Co-ordinator SIVA
Fondazione Pro Juventute
Don Carlo Gnocci
Via Capecelatro 66
20148 Milano
Italy
Tel: +39 2 40308340
Fax: +39 2 26861144

Mr Angelo Paganin
Co-ordinator
Centro Study PRISMA
Fondazione Don Aldo Belli
Via Lucarno 24
1–32 100 Belluno
Italy
Tel/Fax: +39 437 941312

Mr Guiliano De Min
Manager
Centro Study PRISMA
(Contact address as above)

E ZOOT (Canada)

Mr John Mitchell
Supervisor
Youth Prevention Program
Alberta Alcohol and Drug Abuse Commission
803 Energy Square Building
10109–106 Street
Edmonton
Alberta TJ5 3L7
Canada
Tel: +1 403 427-4267
Fax: +1 403 427-0456

Electronic alarms

Canada

Ms Elizabeth Tondu
Director
Good Samaritan Lifeline
9649–71 Avenue
Edmonton
Alberta T6E 5J2
Canada
Tel: +1 403 4396619

The Netherlands

Mr FJM Vlaskamp
Revalidatie Informatie Centrum
Postbus 88
6430 AB Hoensbroek
Zandsbergsweg 111
6432 CC Hoensbroek
Netherlands
Tel: +31 45 239360/239369

Videotelephony

Germany

Mr Thomas Erkert
EMPIRICA
Gesellschaft fur Kommunikations-und Technologie Forschung MBH
Oxfordstrasse 2
D–5300 Bonn 1
Germany
Tel: +49 228 98 530-0
Fax: +49 228 98 530-12

Portugal

Ms Maria Pereira A Martins
CET Centro de Escudos de Telecommunicoes
Rua Eng. Jose Ferreira Pinto Basto
P 3800 Aveiro
Portugal
Tel: +351 34 20101
Fax: +351 34 20722

Public participation in decision making

Canada

Mr MJ Hollingshead
President
Facing the Future Inc.
15003–56 Avenue
Edmonton
Alberta T6H 5B7
Canada
Tel: +1 403 438-7342
Fax: +1 403 434-7451

USA

Ms Ann Sheehan
Executive Director
Berks Community Television
645 Penn Street
Reading
PA 19601
USA
Tel: +1 215 374-3065

Glossary of Abbreviations

AADAC	Alberta Alcohol and Drug Abuse Commission (Canada)
APPSN	Application Pilot for People with Special Needs (RACE programme)
AIM	Advances in Informatics in Medicine (now Telematics in Health Care)
BBS	(Electronic) Bulletin Board System
BCTV	Berks Community Television (Reading, USA)
BIRD	Better Infrastructure for Rural Development (RACE programme)
CD-ROM	Compact Disc for data storage
ENIL	European Network for Independent Living
EPIC	European Prototype for Integrated Care
ETM	Electronic Town (hall) Meeting
E ZOOT	Electronic bulletin board for youth health promotion
FASDE	Future Alarm and Awareness Services for the Disabled and Elderly
HANDYNET	A HELIOS project to establish a Europe wide information system on living with disability
HELIOS	Handicapped People in the European Community Living in an Open Society. An EC action programme to promote educational, occupational, economic and social integration, and an independent way of life for disabled people.
HFA	Health for All. Movement initiated by World Health Organization (European region) to reorient service provision to primary health care (see WHO, 1986).
IBC	Integrated Broadband Communications
ISDN	Integrated Services Digital Network
PHC	Primary Health Care

PRS	Personal (alarm) Response Systems
RACE	Research and Development in Advanced Communications Technologies in Europe
TIDE	Technology Initiative for Disabled and Elderly People
VT	Videotelephony (two-way television)
WHO	World Health Organization

References

Agdestein S and Roemer M (1991) Good health at a modest price: the fruit of primary care. *World Health Forum,* **12** (4), 428–31.

Andricht R and Pedotti A (1992) SIVA: *A computerized information network supporting the choice of technical aids in Italy.* Proceedings of the World Congress on Disability, 1–5 December 1991, Washington, USA.

Armstrong D (1993) From clinical gaze to regime of total health. In: Beattie A, Gott M, Jones L and Sidell M (eds) *Health and wellbeing: A Reader.* Macmillan in association with the Open University, England.

Ashton J (ed) (1992) *Healthy cities.* Open University Press, Milton Keynes, England.

Ashton J and Seymour H (1988) *The New Public Health: the Liverpool Experience.* Open University Press, Milton Keynes, England.

Ballabio E, Placencia-Porrero I and Puig de la Bellacasa R (eds) (1993) Videotelephony support for elderly people. In: *Rehabilitation technology: strategies for the European Union.* IOS Press, Amsterdam, The Netherlands.

Beattie A (1988) *Knowledge and Control in Health Promotion.* Paper given at King's Fund Conference on Sociology of the Health Service: contemporary problems, 2 December 1988, London, England.

Beattie A, Gott M, Jones L and Sidell M (eds) (1993) *Health and Wellbeing: a reader.* Macmillan Press, London, England.

Biag S (1991) *Telematics in primary health care.* Keynote address, workshop proceedings, 21–22 June 1991, AIM Central Office, Brussels, Belgium.

Bougie T (1991) *The Dutch system for providing technical aids to individual users: Marketing and purchasing systems.* Rehabilitation engineering technology, pp 93–8. Proceedings, 2nd workshop on rehabilitation engineering, 12–15 May 1991, Fagernes, Norway.

Boydell L (1992) Home is where the health is. *British Journal of Healthcare Computing,* July, p 16.

Broughton W (1991) Qualitative methods in program evaluation. *American Journal of Health Promotion,* **5** (6), 461–5.

Burnett M (1978) *Endurance of life: the implications of genetics for human life.* Melbourne University Press, Australia.

Callaghan D (1993) Ends and means are one in the quest for survival with dignity. *World Health Forum,* **14**, 126–7.

Carroll L (1865) *Alice in Wonderland* (1st edition). Macmillan, London, England.

Castanheira JL (1991) Promoting the health of adolescents: are we on the right track? *International Journal of Adolescent Medicine and Health,* **5** (2), 113–25.

CDHH&CS (1993) *Goals and targets for Australia's health in the year 2000 and beyond.* Department of Public Health, University of Sydney, Australia.

CEC (1993) *AIM research and development action workplan 1991–94.* Commission of the European Communities, Brussels, Belgium.

CEC (1993) *Commission communication on the framework for action in the field of public health.* COM (93)559, Commission of the European Communities, Brussels, Belgium.

CEC (1993) *Fourth framework programme for community research and technical development 1993–98.* COM (93)459, Commission of the European Communities, Brussels, Belgium.

CEC (1993) *TIDE 1993–94 workplan.* Commission of the European Communities, Brussels, Belgium.

Clausen J (1992) Midwifery in Denmark, MIDIRS Midwifery Digest, **2** (3), 267–8.

Cullan K and Moran R *et al.* (1991) *Technology and the elderly: the role of technology in prolonging the independence of the elderly in the community care context*. Research report FOP 296 funded under Forecasting and Assessment in Science and Technology (FAST) programme of the Commission of the European Communities, Brussels, Belgium.

Cunningham R (1992) *Promoting better health in Canada and the USA*. Department of Politics, University of Glasgow, Scotland.

Dalton KJ and Currie J (1986) Home telemetry made simple. *Journal of Obstetrics and Gynaecology*, **6**, 151–4.

Dawson AJ, Middlemiss C, Jones EM and Gough NAJ (1988) Fetal heart rate monitoring by telephone: **1** Development of an integrated system in Cardiff. *British Journal of Obstetrics and Gynaecology*, October 1988, **95**, 1018–23.

Donabedian A (1980) *Explorations in quality assessment and monitoring*. Volume 1. Health Administration press, Ann Arbor, Michigan, USA.

Donabedian A (1982) *Explorations in quality assessment and monitoring*. Volume 2. Health Administration Press, Ann Arbor, Michigan, USA.

Donabedian A (1985) *Explorations in quality assessment and monitoring*. Volume 3 . Health Administration Press, Ann Arbor, Michigan, USA.

Dripps JH, Boddy K and Venters G, (1992) Telemedicine: requirements standards and applicability to remote care scenarios in Europe. In: Van Goor JN and Christensen JP, (eds) *Advances in medical informatics*, pp 340–8. Results of an AIM exploratory action, IOS Press, Amsterdam, Oxford, Washington DC, Tokyo.

D'Souza M (1992) *The theoretical basis behind screening*. Paper given at Royal Society of Medicine conference, 14 September 1992, London, England.

Dutton DB (1988) *Worse than the disease: pitfalls of medical progress*. Cambridge University Press, England.

Ebeling K and Nischan P (1992) Nonexperimental evaluation of the effectiveness of a screening programme for lung cancer. *International Journal of Technology Assessment in Healthcare*, **8** (2), 245–54.

Erkert T (1992) Elderly persons and communications. In: Bouma H and Graafmans J, (eds) *Gerontechnology*, pp 293–303. IOS Press, Amsterdam, The Netherlands.

Erkert T, De Graat T and Robinson S (1993) *Der haus – tele dienst in Frankfurt am main, projektbericht*. Kuratorium Deutsche Altershilfe, Koln, Germany.

Etzioni A (1993) *The spirit of community: rights, responsibilities, and the communitarian agenda*. Crown, New York, USA.

Feyerband P (1975) *Against method.* Verso, London, England.

Gann R (1991) Progress in documentation and consumer health information: the growth of an information specialism. *Journal of Documentation,* **47** (3), 284–308.

Gelijne AC and Halm EA (1991) *Medical innovation at the crossroads.* Volume 2: *The changing economics of medical technology.* National Academy Press, Washington DC, USA.

Gibbins R L, Riley M and Brimble P (1993) Effectiveness of a programme for reducing cardiovascular risk for men in one general practice. *British Medical Journal,* **306**, 1652–6.

Giles WD and Lewis R (1992) Influencing corporate direction: a case study from British Telecom. *Marketing Intelligence and Planning,* **10** (4), 23–35.

Godinho J, Rathwell T, Gott M and Daley J (1991) *Tipping the balance towards primary healthcare,* p 275. Final scientific report of the research project of the Commission of the European Communities, Brussels, Belgium.

Godinho J, Rathwell T, Gott M, Giraldes R and Daley J (1992) Tipping the balance. *European Journal of Public Health,* **2** (3 & 4), special issue.

Gott M and O'Brien M (1990) *The role of the nurse in health promotion: policies, perspectives and practice.* Department of Health, London, England.

Gott M and Packham H (1993) The quality of community nursing services: report of an exploratory study in a UK health authority. *International Journal of Health Care Quality Assurance,* **6** (1), 24–31.

Green LW (1991) Everyone has a theory, few have measurement. *Health Education Research,* **6** (2), 249–50.

Greenland S (1990) *Science versus public health action: those who were wrong are still wrong.* Invited commentary, Department of Epidemiology, UCLA School of Public Health, Los Angeles, USA.

Hancock T (1992) News from the planet Pandora. In: van Berlo A and Kiwitz de Ruijter Y (eds) *A healthy society – health in the information society,* pp 295–302. Akontes Publishing, Knegsel, The Netherlands.

Hansen WB and Graham JW (1991) Preventing alcohol, marijuana and cigarette use among adolescents: peer pressure resistance training versus establishing conservative norms. *Preventative Medicine,* **20**, 414–30.

Henderson H (1993) *Redefining wealth and progress.* Paper given at Healthy Cities and Communities conference, 8–11 December 1993, San Francisco, USA.

Hill WC, Fleming DA and Martin RW *et al.* (1990) Home uterine activity monitoring is associated with a reduction in preterm birth. *Obstetrics and Gynaecology,* **76** (1), (supplement), 13–18.

HMSO (1992) *Maternity services* (Winterton report). 2nd report and Proceedings of the Health committee. House of Commons, Volume 1, HMSO, London, England.

Humphreys A (1992) HANDYNET European information system: rhetoric or reality? *Assignation,* **9** (2), 48–51.

Hutton J (1991) Medical device innovation and public policy in the European Economic Community. In: Gelijns AC and Halm EA *Medical innovation at the crossroads (Volume 2): The changing economics of medical technology.* National Academy Press, Washington, DC, USA.

IHCFF (1988) *A view of the horizon.* Institute for Health Care Facilities of the Future. Ottawa, Canada.

IRV (1990) *Alarm systems for the elderly and disabled.* Institute for Rehabilitation Research, Hoensbroek, The Netherlands.

IRV (1990) *Some background information about the system in the Netherlands.* Paper given at the First International Symposium on Emergency Response Services for Frail Persons Living Alone, May 1990, Washington DC, USA.

Jackson J (1992) *Electronic ZOOT annual report, 1992.* AADAC Community Education Service, Edmonton, Alberta, Canada.

Jackson J (1993) *Exploring Computer-mediated communication structures on an electronic bulletin board: a unique context for anonymous interaction.* Department of Sociology, University of Alberta, Edmonton, Canada.

Jacobson B, Smith A and Whithead M (eds) (1991) *The nation's health: a strategy for the 1990s.* King's Fund, London, England.

Johnson M (1990) Natural sociology and moral questions in nursing: can there be a relationship? *Journal of Advanced Nursing,* **15**, 1358–62.

Jones AL (1990) *Non-technological factors and perspectives: EURODIABETA modelling and implementation of information systems for chronic healthcare – example: diabetes.* Report of AIM project (A1019), Commission of the European Communities, Brussels, Belgium.

Jonkers-Kuiper L (1992) Knowledge management and community involvement. In: van Berlo A and Kiwitz de Ruijter Y (eds) *A healthy society – health in the information society*. Akontes Publishing, Knegsel, The Netherlands.

Konner M (1993) *The trouble with medicine*. BBC Books, London, England.

Leadbetter N (ed) (1992) *European health services handbook*. Institute of Health Services Management, London, England.

Lefebvre CR (1991) Promoting health promoters: professional development in health promotion. *Health Promotion International*, **6** (1), 1–2.

Middlemiss C, Dawson AJ, Gough N, Jones E, and Coles EC (1989) A randomized study of a domiciliary antenatal care scheme: maternal psychological effects. *Midwifery*, **5**, 69–74.

Milio N (1986) Telematics in the future of health care delivery: implications for nursing. *Journal of Professional Nursing*, January to February.

Milio N (1990) The press and policy making: clues for creating a health promoting climate. *International Quarterly of Community Health Education*. **10** (4), 329–346.

Milio N (1992) New tools for community involvement in health. *Health Promotion International*, **7** (3), 209–17.

Ministry of Health, Welfare and Cultural Affairs (Netherlands) (1992) *Choices in health care*. Zoetermeer, The Netherlands.

Myers A (1987) Anonymity is part of the magic. In: Jackson J (1993) *Exploring computer-mediated communication structures on an electronic bulletin board: a unique context for anonymous interaction*. Department of Sociology, University of Alberta, Edmonton, Canada.

National Information Infrastructure (1993) Agenda for Action. *Inside Multimedia*, **78** (supplement), 30 December 1993, 1–12.

Newell (1993) *Conference report*. InterCHI Conference, April 1993 Amsterdam, The Netherlands.

NIFI (1992) *The healthcare Crisis: containing costs, expanding coverage*. National Issues Forums Institute, Dayton, Ohio, USA.

Nutbeam D, Aaro L and Wold B (1991) The lifestyle concept and health education with young people. Results from a WHO international survey. *Journal of the Institute of Health Education*, **29** (3), 98–103.

OECD (1988) *Ageing populations: the social policy implications.* Organizations for Economic Co-operation and Development, Paris, France.

OECD (1992) *Cities and new technologies.* Organization for Economic Co-operation and Development, Paris, France.

Omerod P (1994) *The death of economics.* Faber, London, England.

Osborne D and Gaebler T (1993) *Reinventing government: how the entrepreneurial spirit is transforming the public sector.* Plume, Penguin, USA.

OTA (1991) *Rural America at the crossroads: networking for the future.* Congress of the United States, Office of Technology Assessment, Washington DC, USA.

Pietroni P (1993) The return of the spirit. In: Beattie A *et al.* (1993) *Health and Wellbeing: a reader,* pp 303–10. Macmillan Press, London, England.

Premiers Commission (1989) *The rainbow report: our vision for health.* Board of Health, Alberta, Canada.

RACE (1993) *Evaluation of the service pilots.* Application Pilots for People with Special Needs (RACE 1054), RACE Project Office, Brussels, Belgium.

Robinson S (1992) Support for Elderly People using Videotelephony. In: Bouma H and Graafmans J (eds) *Gerontechnology,* pp 305–16. IOS Press, Amsterdam, The Netherlands.

Roger France FH and Santucci G (1991) *Perspectives on information processing in medical applications: strategic issues, requirements and options for the European Community.* Springer-Verlag, Berlin, Germany.

Roling D (1992) The citizen's view. In: van Berlo A and Kiwitz de Ruijter Y (eds) *A healthy society – health in the information society,* pp 11–16. Akontes Publishing, Knegsel, The Netherlands.

Rosen M and Lindholm L (1992) The neglected effects of lifestyle interventions in cost-effectiveness analysis. *Health Promotion International,* 7 (3), 163–9.

Sax S (1990) *Healthcare choices and the public purse.* Allen and Unwin, Sydney, Australia.

Schofield J (1993) *All on a silver platter.* Computer review, 28 January, Guardian Newspapers, London, England.

Siler-Wells (1988) Public participation in community health. *Health Promotion (Canada),* **27** (1), 7–11, 23.

Stuurop K (1992) Information is only meaningful in a process of communication. In: van Berlo A and Kiwitz de Ruijter Y (eds) *A healthy society – health in the information society*, pp 51–6. Akontes Publishing, Knegsel, The Netherlands.

Tagawa O (1992) The wise women of France. MIDIRS Midwifery Digest, **2** (2), 136–8.

Teijlingen ER (1989) Going Dutch? *Midwife, Health Visitor and Community Nurse*, **25** (4), 146–7.

Tetzchner S von (1991) (ed) *Issues in telecommunication and disability*. (COST 219). DG Telecommunications, Information Industries and Innovation, Commission of the European Communities, Luxembourg.

Toussaint J (1991) Midwifery in Germany: part 1. *MIDIRS Midwifery Digest*, **1** (1), 15–16.

UNICEF/WHO (1992) *Strategies to promote and maintain the healthy development of young people*. Working group report, November 1991. New York, USA.

Van Goor JN and Christensen JP (1992) *Advances in medical informatics: results of the AIM exploratory action*. IOS Press, Amsterdam, The Netherlands.

Veneris Y (1992) *The electronic home: interactive telecommunications of the future and the social impact of telemedicine at home*. Report to European Foundation for the Improvement of Living and Working Conditions, working paper WP/92/12/EN. Dublin, Ireland.

Venters G (1990) *Telemedicine application – An Industry Approach: research and development in medical and bio-informatics*. Report of AIM workshop, 22 October 1990, AIM Central Office, Brussels, Belgium.

Verbraak P (1992) Informing healthcare. In: van Berlo A and Kiwitz de Ruijter Y (eds) *A healthy society – health in the information society*, pp 33–5. Akontes Publishing, Knegsel, The Netherlands.

WHO (1978) *Alma Ata Declaration*. Regional Office for Europe, Copenhagen, Denmark.

WHO (1985) *Targets for Health For All* (revised 1992). Regional Office for Europe, Copenhagen, Denmark.

WHO (1986) *Ottawa Charter*. Regional Office for Europe, Copenhagen, Denmark.

WHO (1993) *Evaluation of recent changes in the financing of health services.* Report of a WHO study group, WHO technical report series 829, Geneva, Switzerland.

Young M and Schuller T (1991) *Life after work: the arrival of the ageless society.* Harper Collins, London, England.

Index